IT'S FAT LOSS, NOT WEIGHT LOSS

IT'S FAT LOSS,

NOT WEIGHT LOSS

The Underground Secret
to Permanent Results

Author Jack T Kunkel M.S. with Dominick M Manfredo

Editor Paul Nandzik

ISBN: 1508972451
ISBN 13: 9781508972457
Library of Congress Control Number: 2015904592
CreateSpace Independent Publishing Platform
North Charleston, South Carolina

Table of Contents

About Jack

Two words that sum up my life story are "drive" and "dedication."

GROWING UP

Nothing in life seemed to come easy for me. My parents went through a messy divorce when I was two years old; I grew up in a bad neighborhood; I was diagnosed with dyslexia in first grade, which crippled my self-confidence and made me feel dumb; and I was so uncoordinated that I needed occupational therapy. I was always comparing myself to people like my sister, who was a genius and an all-star athlete. You can understand why I was mad at the world.

I turned to tobacco, alcohol, drugs and other dangerous activities as the outlet for my pain and frustration. My life spiraled out of control and I'm really blessed to even be alive. After barely graduating high school in 1995, I realized that there was more to life, that I needed to stop feeling sorry for myself and if I didn't make a change now I was going to end up in jail or dead.

I went cold turkey one morning and never went back. One by one I lost so-called "friends" who I thought would be there for me until the very end. But without the partying, we didn't seem to have much in common.

THE GYM BECAME MY LIFE

I chose a new outlet at the gym. I became obsessed with building muscle and studied everything I could find about nutrition and exercise, especially bodybuilding. When the magazines told me to eat 12 eggs, 4 chicken breasts, 8 white potatoes, a cup of oatmeal and rice, well, that's exactly what I did. I had no idea that I was essentially poisoning myself with low-quality food, although I suppose this was a step up from the fast food and processed food that I grew up with.

During the mid-90's I had dreams of becoming a bodybuilder, and I scheduled my life around the gym. No matter how hard I worked out, it was never enough. I was so driven to succeed that I overtrained, which resulted in a subluxed kneecap, micro-fractures in my leg and knee that required major surgery to repair, and losing the use of my left leg for well over a year and a half. In my quest to become a bodybuilder, what I had failed to understand was the amount of drugs that bodybuilders were taking in order to maintain their physiques.

ONE DAY I WAS HEALTHY, NEXT DAY NOT SO MUCH

By 2003 I was working in the family business as a paramedic and wanted to do my first drug-free bodybuilding show. I competed for five years and finally turned professional in 2007. I was featured on bodybuilding.com podcasts, appeared in national magazines, fitness websites and tabloids. However, my life changed shortly after my 15 minutes of fame. One day I woke up with no energy at all, low libido and was suffering from extreme depression! Work was becoming the most stressful aspect of my life, I wasn't getting enough sleep, I was working too much, working out too much, stressing out and not eating quality foods. Week after week I continued falling apart, feeling more tired and depressed and experiencing a lower libido. I may have looked like a professional bodybuilder should, but I was a true mess on the inside.

My physician, and several subsequent specialists who I was referred to, diagnosed me with depression, hypothyroid, low testosterone and adrenaline fatigue, and prescribed pharmaceuticals – or pharmaceuticals with supplements – to "fix" the problem. I didn't want to "take a pill for every ill." I knew there was a better way! But after months with no improvement I felt like I had my back against the wall and finally agreed to take them.

I TOOK CONTROL

The medications weren't working and I knew I needed to find the cure myself since no one was going to fight this sickness except me. Endlessly, I researched the best healthcare professionals in the U.S., Chinese medicine, Ayurvedic medicine, functional medicine and positive psychology. This research became my full-time job and I actually enjoyed it so much that I – the dyslexic, uncoordinated kid – went back to school for Applied Clinical Nutrition. I found that the combination of these disciplines gave me the knowledge and power to eliminate my depression, increase my daily energy and libido while burning fat and building muscle! It was like I found the underground secret to success in life, and since then I've devoted myself to helping my clients meet their own nutritional needs, fitness goals and improve their self-confidence!

This book represents years of dogged research, with methods that get results that I have been able to consistently replicate for myself as well as hundreds and hundreds of clients to become "the best you" they can be. Ultimately, that self-empowering transformation has always been the goal.

Let YOUR revolution begin!

EDUCATION

- M.S., Applied Clinical Nutrition, New York Chiropractic College
- B.S., Empire State College

AWARDS & CERTIFICATION

- ACE Certified Health Coach
- ACE Certified Personal Trainer
- Expert Rating Sports Nutrition Certification
- NESTA Certified Corporate Wellness Coach
- Retired Drug-Free Professional Bodybuilder

Foreword

My name is Dr. Kareem Hamad and I have struggled with my weight for as long as I can remember. Having graduated from medical school, I understood how the body's metabolism works, yet I lacked the understanding of how to eat for health. In turn, I met with various nutritionists and tried different weight loss programs, which I **thought** were good for me. Starting at 275 pounds, I would meet short-term goals on these diets and get down as low as 168 pounds, but for every time my weight would go down it would always rise back up shortly thereafter, and with the weight gain I experienced a lack of energy and lean muscle mass loss. At my "best" I was "skinny-fat," meaning my body fat percentage was high and my lean muscle mass was low. After three years of this, I realized I needed to modify my lifestyle and eat to fuel my body rather than just count calories.

I always felt there was a way to combine my medical knowledge with the knowledge of a nutritionist, and so, at 235 pounds and recovering from a knee surgery, I made an appointment to meet with Jack Kunkel.

Interestingly, Jack's understanding of diet was different from what I was taught in medical school. After meeting and discussing with him, it soon became clear that his proposed program, personalized to my body's unique needs, made the most sense to me out of anything else I'd seen. A personalized program is important because, medically speaking, individuals are not the same - some people have slow metabolisms, while others have fast metabolisms and some people are more sensitive to carbohydrates as compared to others. Combining my medical knowledge with Jack's nutritional knowledge and solid exercise plan, I was able to reach 200 pounds with 6% body fat in less than one year.

Reflecting back and seeing myself as a "skinny-fat guy" at 168 pounds as opposed to now being 200 pounds of lean body mass, I currently understand more about how to eat on a day-to-day basis while being able to live my life without being on a "diet." I **enjoy** the food that I eat – so much that I am looking forward to creating my meals each and every day. In addition, I have learned how to enjoy food **socially** without fear of regaining the weight. Compared to other programs, Jack Kunkel's is not about short-lived results. It is a program built around the principle of achieving lifetime results. The education he provides is so powerful because you carry that knowledge with you forever as you become your own personal nutritionist.

I highly recommend Jack's program as well as the information in this book for anyone seeking to gain insight about their body, how it works and its relationship with food.

Kareem Hamad, M.D.

Introduction

Getting into shape can feel like a distant dream or an impossible task, but with the right tools – an education and a little willpower – it's a far closer reality than you might think. Most popular diets revolve around losing weight but barely any talk about just losing fat, and there's a HUGE difference between the two. Furthermore, most of these diets feature magic pills, processed meal replacement bars/drinks and specialized exercise equipment, all of which are expensive and make big promises on results without demanding a change in your lifestyle or an understanding of how their products work. It's understandable to want immediate results, but going on these crash diets can actually damage your body, including your metabolism, which only makes it more difficult to burn fat. And because they often only look at parts of the problem rather than the big picture, results – if any are achieved at all – are almost always temporary, and the cost of their program can suck your wallet or purse dry.

SYSTEMATIC APPROACH
This book provides a systematic approach to help you crack the code to **permanent** fat loss, a less stressful life, increased happiness, and much more! You will achieve **amazing** results by taking some of this information and implementing it at your own pace into your routine without over-burdening your lifestyle. Understanding the basics of nutrition, benefits of exercise, causes of stress and the root of happiness will provide you with the knowledge to change your life for the long-run.

DIET, EXERCISE AND MORE?

It's pretty commonly accepted across the board that proper nutrition and exercise are two of the main components of a healthy lifestyle and rapid fat loss. Health and wellness is more than just the physical – it's the mental and emotional as well. Good sleep hygiene, effective stress management, a balanced self-image and many other elements are necessary components required to not only create permanent results, but to make them **enjoyable** to attain.

To give you an idea, I have taken the Food Pyramid, restructured it into what I believe is the key portions to ultimate fat loss and called it the Fat Loss Pyramid. Most of your success is going to rely on proper nutrition, secondly on exercising, third on your mindset and fourth on your lifestyle – which will all be taught to you throughout this entire book.

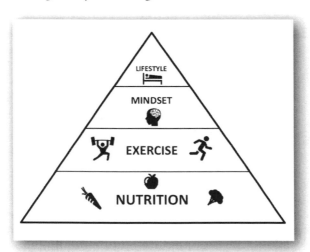

LET'S GET REAL

This book isn't going to sugarcoat anything, and it's not going to provide you with any "quick tricks" to losing inches off your waistline, so if that's what you're looking for, then you need to stop reading and return this book immediately. All this book is doing is simplifying the process for effectively burning fat, creating a healthy long-term lifestyle and providing you with a practical understanding of how some of the science behind health, wellness and fat loss works. Isn't it better to work a little harder ONCE rather than taking shortcut after shortcut and never arriving at the results that you're looking for?

IT'S COMPLICATED BUT WE MAKE IT SIMPLE

Like I said before, everyone knows that exercise and proper nutrition are integral to achieving fat loss and overall health. But it's more complicated than that. Overtraining can cause significant health problems, the quality of the foods you're eating can be drastically affecting the amount of nutrition your body is receiving, and your level of stress can affect your sense of hunger. The list goes on and each chapter of this book goes into detail on all these aspects of health, wellness and more so that you can better understand what drives our bodies to properly function. No more yo-yo dieting, no more deceptions and no more panicking – just a program that will help you achieve your fitness goals step by step.

HARD WORK AND AN EDUCATION

I won't lie – the methods described in this book require dedication, hard work and a willingness to learn. It might not be easy, but every journey begins with a single step and even if you "only" implement this program into your lifestyle little by little you'll still achieve long lasting benefits. And better yet, each chapter starts off with a chart that breaks down that aspect of permanent fat loss by its level of difficulty, how long it takes to implement that step and how important that step is to your overall health.

YOU'RE ONLY AS STRONG AS YOUR WEAKEST LINK

You'll find that some steps are going to be easier than others. And, for example, if you're already getting a great night's sleep, then skip that chapter (for now) for another health aspect that you're having trouble with. Everyone has different strengths, weaknesses and needs, and I always recommend my clients to focus on whatever aspect they know needs the most improvement. This means you'll probably be reading these chapters "out of order." That's fine – just make sure you still read ALL of the chapters because even if you're getting a good night's sleep, reading the chapter on that subject might provide you with additional tips for getting an EVEN BETTER night's sleep!

This book is meant to empower you to make the **right** choices that will help you lose fat **and** become a permanently healthy individual, but only **you** have the power to change - not a practitioner or anyone else.

So what are you waiting for? Get ready, get set and let's get started!

Lifestyle Scale	DESCRIPTION
Serving Size 1 Person Makes 1 Lifetime Result	
Grade Per Person	**Difficulty** - You'll need to **change** your daily habits in order to **repair** a damaged metabolism.
Grade	
Grade*	**Time to Implement** - It takes 1 day to **learn** and 2 days to **start** repairing.
Difficulty 5	
Time to Implement 3 Days	**Importance** - Repairing your metabolism is the first step when trying to see **perrmanent** results.
Importance 8	
*Amount is based off of the average person. Your personal results may be higher or lower depending on your specific needs.	

1

Do you have a damaged metabolism?

NO TIME? EAT THIS

Unlike in other countries around the world, obesity is a disease running rampant throughout America at an unfathomable rate. It doesn't help that there are fast-food restaurants within walking distance in almost every corner of our country. That's what making money is about though, right? Having the ease of convenience and receiving large quantities of food for almost nothing. I don't know about you, but more money in my pockets doesn't necessarily make up for the added inches around my waistline. The biggest problem is that "dining," has become a term of the past. With the high intensity, fast-paced environment that we live in, nobody has time to "dine" anymore. So this term has fallen off the map and been replaced with "convenience food." This convenience food is a low-quality, SOMETIMES low calorie, nutrient deficient food that exists all around us that we can shove into our faces in a moment when we are short on time.

*More than two-thirds of U.S adults are overweight or obese.[1]

Since most of us are too short on time to even properly eat – one of our required bodily functions – we, as a society, have tried our hardest to find the solution to our weight problems the same way: through convenient, easy, low-quality methods.

A CALORIE IS A CALORIE IN A LAB, BUT NOT IN YOUR BODY

BOTH the obesity epidemic and calorie counting started in the 1970s. Is this a coincidence? I think not! The truth behind the "Calories In, Calories Out" rule is way outdated, but not completely worthless. People need to wake up and understand that we become the food we eat, period! Food quality has been all but forgotten in place of food quantity. This is where people are really hurting themselves because foods are not just vitamins and minerals. They are also phytonutrients, energy and information (which will be explained in further detail)! The whole information part is what's going to play a major role in determining your health in the long-run. Processed foods in general, lack nutritional value because they are taken out of their natural state. Most often, there is food out there that **appears** to be healthy, but it is grown in depleted soil with unnatural fertilizers, making it nutrient deficient!

*Natural State - a wild original state unprocessed by people.

Quality is not the whole issue though. Quantity can also be the problem. Just for example, I like to use 2,000 calories per day of quality foods as the norm for the average person, which is just a baseline metabolic rate. Your metabolic rate typically falls in a range of 500 calories from your calorie set point. If you consume 500 more calories per day, this will lead to **a gain in body fat**, but if you were to consume 500 fewer calories per day, this will lead to **a loss in body fat**. Now, everyone is different, whether you have a sedentary job like sitting at a desk, or you might be a carpenter moving regularly. These two lifestyles make a big difference in your metabolic set point. Your age, how much muscle you have, how well you sleep, how much stress you endure each day, the type and amount of medication you take and the health of your gut bacteria are all factors that affect your metabolism. And there's even more that I will get into. I know taking this all in can be overwhelming, but this is why I want to teach you in a systematic, non-threatening way to help you understand what works for you and your personal lifestyle.

*Set point - the body's thermostat for the regulation of body fat and weight, which is unique.

*If you are choosing quality foods, you will naturally eat less.

FASTER METABOLISM RESULTS IN FASTER FAT LOSS

Your metabolism is one of the most important bodily functions for losing body fat. It's responsible for either **massive** results or an **enormous** flop. But why? Well, first of all, metabolisms are different for everyone, so we must look at fat loss on an individual, case-by-case basis. Depending on your current height, weight and eating habits, your metabolic range could be different compared to friends or family. And, believe it or not, you can even be eating the same exact amount and type of food as one of your training buddies, friends or family members, but still have different results.

I always see on television how females have more trouble losing weight compared to males, and this might be one of the only truthful facts that we are given through the media. Females usually have an average metabolic rate 5% to 10% lower than males do. This is because females naturally have more body fat on their frames, which protects their vital organs if they were to become pregnant. This increased amount of body fat results in a lower metabolic rate because they have less lean muscle than the typical male. This doesn't mean that you women should give up and call it quits. Just because it's going to be a tougher road doesn't mean that it will never happen. The results that you will see when you do everything the right way will **blow your mind**. Not only will you look better, but you will also FEEL better!

FAT LOSS ONLY PLEASE

The ultimate goal for permanent fat loss lies in losing body fat, not just "weight" in general. Hence, the book title, *It's Fat Loss, Not Weight Loss: The Underground Secret to Permanent Results*. This seems like a no-brainer, but the truth is that so many people are dieting the wrong way, leading to the wrong type of "weight" loss. You are probably saying to yourself, "There is a bad type of weight loss?" That's right! Not all "weight" loss is good, especially if it's not done in the proper way. The key to permanent weight loss is to maintain or gain lean muscle while torching off body fat. Why lean muscle? Well, one pound of resting lean muscle burns around 10 calories a day![2, 3] So this means that our goal is to create lean muscle on your frame that will aid in your fat loss. The more lean muscle you have on your frame, the higher your metabolism, the more calories you burn just by performing your daily activities.

FAD DIETS: LOSE FAST, GAIN IT BACK FASTER

In addition, your metabolism, like any other system of your body, can be damaged if not taken care of. Many dieters have succumbed to the world of fad dieting. Commonly, fad dieters are provided with **no education** and **biased information,** which ultimately results in a **damaged metabolism**.

When you turn on the TV in the morning and scroll through the channels, you can see that many people are hopping on the fad diet bandwagon, which results in a vicious circle of diet after diet, commonly referred to as "yo-yo dieting." There's "The Fix," "Lose Weight by Eating 500 Calories" and the "Don't Eat Anything But Our Shakes" diets bombarding our brains.

The worst part about most of these diets is that they can actually put you further behind than when you first started! When you are going on one of these fad diets, your metabolism will shut down because your body doesn't know that you are starving it on purpose. A high metabolism will burn body fat and use up energy, but since your body thinks it's being starved, it will try to use up the driving force of your metabolism, which is your **muscle**. Since your body is trying to slow its metabolism down, it will use muscle as an energy source instead of fat and glycogen (stored carbohydrates in the muscle and liver). Muscle is an insufficient energy source for your body, which can cause many more problems down the road. Your muscle has a lot of not-so-efficient amino acids that your body is using, leaving you nutrient deficient and, eventually, making you more toxic than you were in the first place. Muscle's made up of about 75% water, so when someone goes on a crash fad diet and loses 30lbs in the first 30 days, it's a mixture of muscle, water and not nearly as much fat as they would like.

These diets are not only providing you with no education and giving you temporary results, but they are also HURTING your body by damaging your metabolism. Instead of losing just straight body fat, you are going to be losing little body fat, a lot of muscle and a bunch of water. This is why results are so temporary, because these drastic losses lead your body to recover by storing fat as a safety mechanism.

*Water makes up more than half our bodyweight; every single cell depends on it, and your metabolism will decrease without it! [4]

THE MAGIC PILL: IF THERE WERE ONE, WE WOULD ALL TAKE IT

So, why are we still falling into the trap? Well, it's definitely hard to pass up a "magic pill" that sheds weight, but not necessarily fat, without having to change your lifestyle. The reality is that you AREN'T becoming healthier by taking these pills. If it sounds like it's a scam, then in all likelihood, it probably is. Just as Rome wasn't built in a day, neither will your dream body. Instead, by giving your body a healthy foundation, month by month, you ARE going to get better. So sticking to your guns and putting in the hard work NOW will lead to lifetime results little by little. Make sure to change the way that you THINK. In a year from now, you could have lost tons of body fat, gained a bunch of lean muscle, and all by doing it the RIGHT way.

MORE FAT LESS MUSCLE

Now, after a diet, you might be looking at the scale saying to yourself, "But I lost (x) amount of weight by using this fad diet." As we just went over, was this good or bad weight that you lost? The difference is going to lie in what happens when you return to your normal eating habits. If you were provided with no education and lost "bad" weight, you will most likely return to normal eating habits and your body WILL put fat back on your frame. And in the most inconvenient places at that. This will result in the infamous oxymoron of being "skinny fat."

Eating a ton of food-like products, as many fad diets instruct, damages your metabolism by lowering thyroid function and lean muscle mass, and causes a change in how your body reacts when it's introduced to real food again[5]. The body is made to adapt, and it wants to be prepared for the next time that a drastic decrease in calorie consumption (e.g., starvation) could happen. Even though your brain knows that you have food available at any time, the body's instincts take over to protect us. In this case by storing fat.

Eating is actually your ally when looking to lose body fat, but choosing quality foods, eating them at the right time and having portion control is the key.

INSULIN RESISTANCE & YOUR METABOLISM

Another big reason why your metabolic rate could be damaged is because of the type of food that you eat. We could have all guessed this by now, but not known why. When someone eats large amount of simple, refined carbohydrates like soda, candy, energy drinks and other sugar-filled foods, this confuses your body on how to regulate your blood-sugar level.

*Insulin - a hormone produced in the pancreas that allows energy to be absorbed into your cells.

After you flood your body with sugar by eating this garbage food, your body uses a natural defense to protect itself against high amounts of sugar by releasing a large amount of insulin into the blood stream. These high levels of insulin down-regulate your metabolism so much that you won't even have a chance to burn fat for energy. If you choose these foods often, the chronically high insulin levels in your blood stream will **not** allow your body to use its own fat for energy.

If you are constantly abusing the system like most people, you will always have insulin floating around in your blood stream – even in between meals. And in between meals is one of the most important times to fight the urge to eat, because that's when you want your insulin levels low, not elevated.

When insulin levels are chronically high, your fat-burning hormones, like glucagon, will not be able to do their job, which is to use that body fat for energy. This is known as **hyperinsulinemia** or **insulin resistance**, and it's my worst nightmare if a client is trying to lose body fat. If you cannot take care of insulin resistance first, you **will not** lose fat. Period! But don't worry – insulin resistance can be taken care of by exercising, changing your diet and practicing my wellness tips!

To give you a mental picture of what occurs when insulin resistance happens, here is my Insulin Resistance Chart:

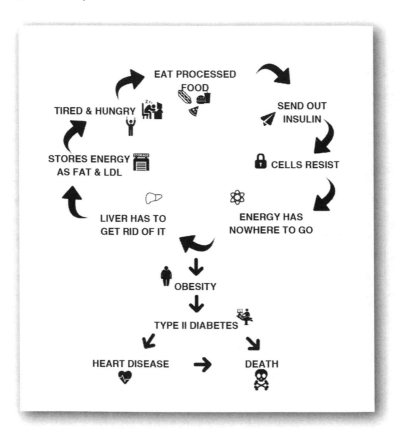

EATING TOO MUCH BUT STILL STARVING?

Having these high amounts of insulin in your system will cause your body to feel that it needs to overeat because your cells still think that they are hungry since they are being starved of good nutrients. Insulin works like a key and lock - the key is insulin, and the lock is the receptors in your cells. When you have insulin resistance, the key no longer fits in the lock, so the energy has no way to get into your cells and so floats around in your bloodstream until your body stores that energy as fat or makes it into bad cholesterol (LDL) to be used at a later date. And after that, low energy follows. The worst part is that when this constantly happens, you aren't ever using that fat for energy "later," but just adding to those reserves for no reason.

MOVE MORE & EAT BETTER, NO PILL REQUIRED

You have to fight the urge to keep reaching for processed foods and foods full of sugar so that you can repair your metabolism. You have to treat your body like a temple and only allow the highest quality foods to enter. When I suspect insulin resistance in my clients, I have the client concentrate on eating high amounts of fiber, healthy fats and proteins. Furthermore, exercising and moving more works just like insulin by activating your energy receptors, called GLUT4, which allows food energy to be absorbed and used by your cells!

The bottom line is that if your metabolism is damaged and if you don't repair it, fat loss is going to be much harder to attain. The good news is that this program is designed to set you up for ultimate success, part of which means repairing your metabolism.

*The Rant: Whether it's damaged from insulin resistance, not training, using fad diets or eating the wrong types of food, you MUST know that fixing your metabolism is the first step in seeing permanent results.

Lifestyle Scale	DESCRIPTION
Serving Size 1 Person Makes 1 Lifetime Result	
Grade Per Person	**Difficulty** - It will not be very hard to **learn** the story behind **real** food.
Grade	
Grade*	**Time to Implement** - It will **only** take you the amount of time to read this chapter.
Difficulty 3	
Time to Implement 1 Day	**Importance** - Without a proper **understanding** of what food really is, **fat loss** may never be achieved.
Importance 9	
*Amount is based off of the average person. Your personal results may be higher or lower depending on your specific needs.	

2

What is food?

Every time science thinks they have it all figured out, mother nature/ higher power/God (or whatever you call it), puts a twist into what people think they know. How many times do pharmaceuticals and supplements get taken off the market? How often do our food recommendations keep changing? This is just plain old confusing, and at times, pretty unethical! All of these are partially the reason why obesity rates have skyrocketed in the past decade. Now, you should know that food gives you energy, vitamins and minerals (to be vague), but there's way more to the story, which science may never fully understand.

FOOD SCIENCE
On March 1, 1905, a 26 year-old patent clerk named Albert Einstein proved that everything is made up of energy through his theory of relativity,

$E=mc^2$. Everything in the universe is made up of energy, including **every** cell and **every** atom in your body. These atoms are made up of 99.99999% energy and only 00.00001% physical substance. Therefore, choosing quality foods that provide you with good energy will increase both your health and metabolism for the long-run.

Stanford School of Medicine Institute for Stem Cell Biology and Regenerative Medicine division explains, "Every one of us completely regenerates our own skin every 7 days. A cut heals itself and disappears in a week or two. Every single cell in our skeleton is replaced every 7 years." What gives you the energy and nutrients in order to do this? Food. Your body breaks down every piece of food that you eat and makes it a part of you! If you eat something that is alive like a salad, it's a "live food," which creates health and life from within; increasing your metabolism and accelerating fat-loss. What happens if you eat a processed "food-like product" like a bag of chips? Well, it's lifeless because of its poor quality, old age, and exposure to heat and oxygen! You should know that lifeless, processed foods impede healing and actually damage your body.

*Lifeless - devoid of any living energy and nutrients. I think of a can of tuna that is 2 years old compared to fresh tuna that's two days old.

YOU CALL THAT FOOD?
When I refer to some foods as "food-like products" it's because they're processed to a point where many experts believe that they technically shouldn't be classified as food anymore.

When you break it all down, these "food-like products" really are old and/or altered foods with poor quality that cause your healthy metabolism to downgrade at a rapid rate! This just makes it so much harder to recover and repair your metabolism, but it's definitely still possible.

In addition, these "food-like products" could have been genetically modified organisms (GMO) in laboratories and deemed safe to consume by food "experts." Unbelievable, I know, but it's happening **everywhere** around us. The American Academy of Environmental Medicine released a position paper stating that "GMO foods pose a serious health risk."[1] The Food and Drug Administration (FDA) approved the first GMO in 1982. Since they have only been around for such a short period of time, the long-term effects have yet to be determined, begging the question, are these foods actually safe to eat? Personally, I will not touch them, so I recommend the same to you!

Think About This: Currently, there are 26 countries that classify GMOs as illegal.[2] The United States is NOT one of them.

FOOD STORIES
Imagine being a cow in a factory farm with thousands of others, crammed into a tiny space, never seeing the light of day, fed the incorrect types of food like genetically modified corn and processed soy (both cause inflammation), pumped with hormones to accelerate growth and drinking water that is polluted with antibiotics that harm your gut microbiome. What type of information is that cow passing along to your genes? Like every human, every food has a story to tell. As humans, if we were put into these same conditions, we would become extremely weak and ill, which is exactly what is happening to these animals. What we eat becomes us, so choosing a strong, healthy source of food will only benefit your body by providing it good energy and information.

*Gut microbiome - the communal genomes of microorganisms that reside in the gastrointestinal system, which is directly related to our health and metabolism.

This is just another reason why I harp so much on **quality**, because every piece of food you put in your mouth is energy and information transferred into your body. Choosing quality foods will provide you with quality energy, orchestrating a healthy molecular message to **every** cell in your body, providing the tools for a plethora of health benefits such as fat loss, increased strength and more energy!

Now, when choosing your food, think "real" or "unprocessed" foods, whether they are fresh or frozen, and always ask yourself how old it is. The older the food, the less nutrients it has. Therefore, you should always opt for locally grown and raised foods, which are best. Frozen food can, in fact, be flash frozen immediately when it's ready to be harvested. So believe it or not, this means **some** frozen foods can actually be "fresher" than fresh food, but make sure it's **quality** food. You can tell if the frozen produce is high quality by searching for a USDA Organic stamp on the package.

*Real food - food that came from Mother Nature, which provides you with all the energy and nutrients your body needs in order to sustain health; nothing that is manmade or artificial.

*Fresh food - food that is not preserved, tampered with, dehydrated, frozen or smoked.

*The Rant: No matter how you look at it, quality is #1 when referring to your food.

Lifestyle Scale	DESCRIPTION
Serving Size 1 Person Makes 1 Lifetime Result	
Grade Per Person	**Difficulty** - It will not be very hard to **learn** the story behind **real** food.
Grade	
Grade*	**Time to Implement** - It will only take you the amount of time to read this chapter.
Difficulty 3	
Time to Implement 1 Day	**Importance** - Knowing what **real food** is remains vital in this program.
Importance 9	
*Amount is based off of the average person. Your personal results may be higher or lower depending on your specific needs.	

3

Macronutrients: the comprehensive breakdown

Macronutrients (Macros) is just another word for the three main nutrients your body needs: carbohydrates, proteins and fats. I not only want you to read about these vital nutrients in their corresponding sections, but I want you to **understand** them. This will help you to grasp why you are or aren't seeing the results you want.

CARBOHYDRATES
At 4 calories per gram, carbohydrates are the body's main source of energy. Highly active individuals such as athletes and construction workers burn more calories per day, and so need greater quantities of carbs. The best

source of energy dense carbohydrates are found in vegetables and fruits. Other, less ideal, sources can be found in starchy foods like potatoes and grains, but also in legumes and dairy, which are high in calories.

VEGETABLES - THE MOST NUTRIENT DENSE FOOD ON THE PLANET

Plant-based nutrition, especially green vegetables, are calorie for calorie the most nutrient-dense foods on the planet, so people who have vast nutritional deficiencies will benefit greatly from increasing their intake of vegetables. Vegetables are an especially excellent source of carbohydrates for people trying to lose fat because they are packed with dietary fibers that are critical to metabolic activity. They also increase gastrointestinal health by feeding the good bacteria, which increases your metabolism and controls hunger by filling your stomach up both physically and mentally. Dietary fibers pass through the gastrointestinal tract to assist in the removal of waste by attaching to toxins and excreting them out of the body, which helps reduce the risk of multiple chronic diseases.

*Toxins – a poison or chemical that causes bodily harm.

Try eating local or organic fresh vegetables and fruits. I highly recommend that you, "Eat the rainbow," when it comes to veggies because multiple colors are going to represent different phytonutrients that your body needs. These phytonutrients are natural chemicals that can help prevent disease and keep your body functioning at the highest level possible. When looking at different colors, choose green, red, blue/purple, white and yellow/orange vegetables. More than 25,000 phytonutrients are found in plant foods, which is why eating a variety of them will guarantee a benefit to your health. Common phytonutrients that may ring a bell are flavonoids, carotenoids, lignans and resveratrol.

Phytonutrients are known to attack harmful free radicals, lower the risk of certain cancers, reduce inflammation and more! When looking at individual colors, each correlates to different aspects of health. Take yellow and orange vegetables for example, which keep your immune system working properly, and are needed for eye health. However, as you know, we aren't here just for eye health, which is why eating a wide variety of these foods is going to give you the best overall health results.

*Free radicals - uncharged molecules missing an electron, which cause damage to important cellular components (DNA, cell membranes, etc.) when they come in contact with each other.

"Going Green," whether it's by land or sea, is the #1 choice you can make for your body. No, I don't mean recycling and planting trees, but more like eating plant-based nutrition. Green plant-based foods have the highest nutrient density compared to any other. Furthermore, it also has the most amount of chlorophyll, a pigment that allows our red blood cells to function more efficiently!

When thinking green plant-based nutrition, some choices are:

- Swiss chard
- Mustard greens
- Spinach
- Bok choy
- Watercress
- Beet greens
- Kale
- Arugula
- Broccoli
- Brussels sprouts
- Wheatgrass
- Parsley
- Basil
- Cilantro

- Nori (kelp)
- Spirulina (algae)
- Chlorella (algae)

Eating salads, baking or grilling veggies are not only extremely nutritious and filling, but you can make them incredibly delicious. I always add green vegetables to a smoothie each day as a great way to sneak in some extra nutrients. Green leafy vegetables like kale works perfect for this, and the best part is that they don't overpower the flavor of the drink. The green color of these shakes doesn't look very appealing, but the taste and nutrients you are going to receive will be worth getting over the looks. This is especially true after we learn to retrain our taste buds from the intense amount of flavor enhancers (e.g., MSG, sugar, salt and fat) contained in "food-like products" people have been consuming for years!

RAW VS. COOKED

Believe it or not, it makes a difference when you are choosing to eat vegetables raw vs. cooked. When you cook foods on the grill, bake them in the oven or microwave them, you are depleting many of the food's natural vitamins, minerals and phytonutrients. The heat (specifically anything above 115°F) essentially destroys the enzymes, which are proteins that accelerate metabolic reactions in the body. So by eating your veggies raw, you are preserving so many of these good enzymes for your body to use. Major healing centers like the Hippocrates Health Institute have been using raw vegetables to increase the amount of enzymes in the body, which helps reverse or even cure diseases. However, you must keep in mind that we are talking **plant-based** nutrition here, so the same may not be safe to ingest when we are talking about other types of food like meats.

You don't have to eat raw veggies exclusively, but putting more into your body will bring you tremendous health benefits, especially considering there are well over 3,000 enzymes that are needed in order for your metabolism, digestive tract and immune system to properly function.[1]

The easiest way to "sneak" raw vegetables into your diet is through a smoothie or large salad. If you have gastrointestinal issues like I.B.S., juice the vegetables, but remember that you are stripping the fiber from the foods when you do this. Additionally, eating some raw fruit, nuts and seeds will provide your body with smaller amounts of enzymes.

*Juicing vs. blending – by using a juicer, you are extracting only the juice from the fruit or vegetable NOT the fiber. By blending the fruit or vegetable, you are incorporating the entire food including both juice and fiber.

If you get tired of your routine, get a little outside of your comfort zone by trying some **different** vegetables with your meals. They not only taste great, but they are also stocked with an immense amount of fiber that will curb your appetite in a healthy way. Adding vegetables is absolutely critical for a healthy diet. Try some sweet potatoes, carrots, beets, garlic, onions, bell peppers, cauliflowers, winter squashes, and eggplants. The possibilities to create great tasting, healthy meals are endless!

"Eat food. Not too much. Mostly plants." – Michael Pollan

Vegetables are definitely vital when it comes to losing fat, but what else is classified as plant-based nutrition? Besides vegetables, there are fruits, whole grains, beans, seeds, nuts, spices and herbs.

NATURE'S CANDY

Although they are higher in sugar content, fruits are the second healthiest compared to veggies. However, the sugar they contain is naturally healthy and the dietary fiber they're packed with helps slow the absorption of that sugar down. David S. Ludwig, MD, PhD published a perspective piece in The Journal of the American Medical Association, which showed an increase in fruit consumption is correlated to lower body weight and lower risk for disease.[2] I recommend a variety of in-season fruits, but my favorites for fat loss are berries, pears and apples for their low sugar content. Keep in mind that the benefits of all fruits in **small amounts** are immeasurable. Personally, my only carbohydrate sources come from vegetables and fruits - I highly recommend you do the same.

DECEPTIVE ADVERTISING

False advertising has people believing that eating grain is essential for fiber and nutrients, but this is not the case. The reason is because of what I like to call "the three-headed monster," being lectins, gluten and phytates.[3, 4, 5] There are very high amounts of all three of these in grains like rye, spelt and wheat. Lectin is a natural anti-nutrient for humans because they bind to the human intestinal lining to cause inflammation and a lower metabolism. Gluten, found in most processed foods, elevates the body's blood-sugar level quickly. Phytates attach to minerals in the body and make them unavailable for absorption. If you must ingest any type of grain, non-gluten grains like brown rice and quinoa are better choices.

*Anti-nutrients - a term that is used to describe the body's inability to absorb or use essential nutrients like vitamins and minerals.

THIS IS WHY CARBS GET A BAD NAME

The worst carbohydrate sources are the ones that are processed and those that absorb too quickly into the body! As stated by Dr. Mark Hyman in his famous book, *The Blood Sugar Solution*, these "Bad Carbs" lead to insulin resistance, the single most leading factor in weight gain, heart disease, stroke, dementia, cancer and a rapid rate in premature aging.[6] Refined carbohydrates like white rice, white potatoes, bread and pasta are the main food culprits. What many don't understand is that liquid calories such as sports drinks, juices, soda, alcohol and flavored coffee are even worse because they spike blood sugar and lower metabolism by causing insulin resistance! These simple carbohydrates have been the reason why carbs have gotten such a bad rap in past years. We have all heard of no-carb diets and people who have lost weight on them, but then gained it all back in a short period of time. The truth behind carbohydrates is that they have a special place in your diet as long as you choose the RIGHT ones. This WILL be the difference between seeing temporary versus permanent results in the long-run.

SOME EXAMPLES OF CARBS TO AVOID

- Doughnuts
- Candy
- Pastries
- Pretzels
- Packaged granola bars
- Sugar-sweetened, instant oatmeal packets
- Crackers
- Muffins
- Cookies
- Pasta
- Bread
- Cereal
- Snack bars
- Soda
- Any other processed foods

PROTEINS

Also coming in at 4 calories per gram, protein is important because it helps the body grow, aids in tissue repair, produces essential hormones and enzymes and preserves lean muscle mass. You can find the most protein in red meat, poultry, fish and eggs. You can also find smaller amounts in other foods like nuts, beans, organic soy, quinoa, ground flaxseed and chia seed. In addition, there are small amounts of protein in dairy products such as milk, yogurt and cheese, but keep in mind that I do not recommend these protein sources as many people are unaware that they are allergic to them. When digested, proteins are broken down into amino acids. Some of these amino acids are formed in the body naturally and are called nonessential amino acids. The other type, essential amino acids, only gets into our bodies through diet. Now, as with other aspects of diet, I have to emphasize choosing QUALITY proteins as this will aid in fat loss as well as help build lean muscle, which is important in keeping that fat loss permanent!

MEET ME IN THE MIDDLE

I have found that people either don't eat any type of protein at all, or they are overdoing it by A LOT. This is mostly because some people tend to think that they need WAY more protein in their diet than the body actually demands. In addition, other people are "carbaholics," where they think that there is no way in the world that they can eat anything other than carbs. If you are one of these people, do me a favor and meet me in the middle. I am not asking for you to eat protein like a bodybuilder, or to eat it like an herbivore. I am just saying that you should definitely ingest quality proteins and to remember to keep it portion controlled!

I recommended that you have a small portion of a LEAN protein with every meal. A really good example is wild-caught fish from the local fish market. Try free-range, grass-fed and/or organic chicken, pork and red meat. Free-range or organic eggs and soaked beans are also great choices for healthy protein sources. Quality is critical because poor protein sources have stored toxins in their fat cells!

WHY GRASS-FED AND / OR FREE-RANGE?

All of the terms "grass-fed," "free-range," "organic," "hormone-free," "antibiotic-free," etc. seem like they should be a no-brainer when it comes to farming these types of animals. The sad reality is that most animals are no longer fed proper, healthy foods or let out of their cages for five minutes during the day.[7] Most of the meat that you are getting from your grocery store is from farms that treat their animals like garbage.[7] They are stressed out, crammed into tight living corners, pumped full of hormones to increase their size and fed poor quality GMO corn and soy all day long.[7] This process gets that meat from their farm to your plate fast and cost efficiently, but produces poor quality, unhealthy meat. In particular, the hormones and other artificial chemicals added to these poor-quality foods can cause inflammation, which can lead to more health problems and weight gain down the road. Exactly like choosing organic produce, when you choose high-quality meats, in which the animals were treated the right way during their lives, not only is the meat going to taste better, but it will also provide you with the proper nutrition that your body thrives on. In order for you to stay motivated throughout the program, you should switch up the types of meat and always use herbs and spices for flavoring!

HERE ARE A FEW PROTEINS TO AVOID

*Poor quality proteins usually are a result of agriculture industrialization that transforms healthy proteins into unhealthy proteins.

*Also be careful not to overcook meat, fish or poultry due to cancer causing agents.

- Processed meat from fast-food restaurants
- Cold cuts
- Factory farm meats from most grocery stores and restaurants
- Meats in frozen prepared foods
- Hot dogs

YOU HAVE TO EAT IT

What I am really trying to say is that high-quality proteins will provide you with all the essential amino acids, which your body needs in order to create its own, working proteins; low-quality proteins WILL NOT do this. If your current eating habits don't provide you with enough essential amino acids, your cells will begin to break down muscle proteins from your own body to cope with the absence. In addition, they will also start to conserve these essential amino acids by limiting the amount used in protein synthesis – the process of your body using amino acids to make new cells. This is ANOTHER reason why choosing top-quality proteins will help you advance to higher levels of fitness.

NO MEAT? NO WORRIES

Have you ever heard of complimentary proteins? If you aren't a vegetarian or vegan, you probably haven't. When someone consumes proteins like meat, poultry, fish and eggs, they **normally** receive the ample amount of essential amino acids their body needs to properly function. Problems arise when you don't eat these types of protein because, as stated above, your body will start to break down its own protein in order to cope, but since this is a non-efficient source of amino acids, the problem still remains. We get around this problem using something called complementary proteins. When you combine different types of plant-based protein sources, they will complement each other in a way that provides your body with all of the essential amino acids. So when one plant-based source is missing certain essential amino acids, another plant-based source provides it, making the combination a complete protein source.

Really good examples of complementary proteins are legumes and brown rice. Legumes contain two essential amino acids called isoleucine and lysine, but not enough methionine and tryptophan. However, whole grains such as brown rice contain high amounts of methionine and tryptophan, but not enough isoleucine and lysine. Therefore, combining these two foods in a meal will provide your body with four of the essential amino acids, which, in this case, makes these two foods into a complete protein.

FATS

How many of us were taught that fat is public enemy number one? Current research, and time, tells us this is not the case at all! In fact, the obesity epidemic began once we started demonizing fat and replacing it with sugar. We now know that it's sugar, not quality fat, that makes us fat, fast! The facts are stunning. The total number of obese adults 20 years old and over has doubled from 1980 through 2002. The incidence of overweight children and adolescents has tripled.[9]

So coming in at 9 calories per gram, the fear of fat is understandable. However, healthy fats provide energy, growth, development, protect our organs, assist in absorption of certain vitamins and - best of all - they develop your brain. Did I mention that it's one of the three critical nutrients for fat loss (fiber, fat and protein)?

The three types of fats to be aware of are saturated fat, unsaturated fat and trans fat. Both conventional (poor quality) saturated fats, like fats found in meat, lard, butter and cream, and trans fats, like the ones found in fried foods, baked goods and snack foods, have been shown to increase the risk of heart disease and chronic inflammation. These fats are responsible for not only weight gain, but also for all the sickness that follows. Substituting those with quality fats like fatty fish, avocado and organic ghee, has been shown to <u>decrease</u> that risk, but portion control is the key!

REALLY CONFUSING

You should be careful when looking into research done on fat because the information is so different from study to study. The good news is that I am here to tell you the science, not the bias. With all of this contradicting data, who – and what – do we believe? The take-home is this: you can actually ingest fat! What you should be watching out for is not only how much you are ingesting, but also the quality of food that you are choosing. Everyone has heard the saying "quality over quantity," and it's true! However, if you decide to choose a lesser quality meat, you should know that these saturated fats can cause disease! My point is that fats are good when you eat good-quality ones and practice portion control too!

HEALTHY FAT FIRST

When looking for your healthy fats to eat, focus on "quality" fats like omega-3 fatty acids, which are anti-inflammatory. Fishes such as salmon, mackerel, anchovies, sardines and halibut (think S.M.A.S.H.); ground flaxseed, chia seed and pasture raised omega-3 enriched eggs are a few of the **top choices** that contain the highest amount of omega-3 fatty acids. These healthy fats are crucial because the standard American diet is extremely pro-inflammatory.

When choosing your seafood, keep in mind that the smaller the fish the less mercury it may contain. Additionally, opt for wild-caught fish over farm-raised fish since they tend to have less contaminants, no antibiotics and higher amounts of omega-3s. It's the same principle as grass-fed vs. industrial livestock.

However, make sure that you DO NOT get confused by omega-6 fatty acids, **most** of which have been proven to increase inflammation **and** cause weight gain. Omega-3 = good. Omega 6 = bad.

VARIETY IS THE SPICE OF LIFE

It is essential that you eat healthy saturated and unsaturated fats in your diet along with omega-3s by choosing a mixture of any of the following: clarified butter (ghee), coconut butter, avocados, mixed nuts, dark chocolate, cold-pressed extra-virgin olive oil, macadamia nut oil, whole free-range or organic eggs and naturally occurring fats found in quality animal-based protein. All of these will provide your body with the healthy fats that it needs in order to properly function. It will also curb the increase of your blood sugar.

*Your body cannot survive on omega-3 fats alone; you must provide it with a <u>combination</u> of healthy saturated fats, unsaturated fats and omega-3s.

Don't overthink it when it comes to fats, just remember that "quality is king," whether they are saturated or unsaturated. Furthermore, they will aid you in losing that unwanted body fat, but again, portion control still remains extremely important.

TRANS FAT ALERT!

Trans fat and industrial seed oils are the fats that have no place in **anyone's** diet! Trans fats can either be naturally present in food or artificially made. Guess which is worse for you? Artificially made trans fats are created by adding hydrogen to vegetable oil, changing it from an unsaturated fat to a saturated fat. Trans fats are well documented for causing coronary heart disease, increasing "bad cholesterol" (LDL) and decreasing "good cholesterol" (HDL). These types of fats should be avoided at ALL COSTS.

TRANS FAT TO AVOID

- Margarine
- Shortening
- Bisquick
- Cake mixes
- Ramen noodles
- Fast food
- Fries
- Anything deep fried
- Pizza
- Breaded fish sticks
- Pastries
- "Convenience" food
- Frozen prepared food
- Pot pies

The Food and Drug Administration (FDA) allows foods to contain up to 0.5 grams of trans fat per serving and still be to be labeled as having zero grams of trans fat, so always read the ingredients or – even better – just stop eating foods with a label!

The keywords that you should be looking for in the ingredients list that indicate trans fat are:

- Partially hydrogenated
- Hydrogenated
- High stearate
- Stearic-rich

INDUSTRIAL SEED OILS: MAKING SOMETHING HEALTHY UNHEALTHY

Not only do some of these oils have zero anti-inflammatory fat, but they can contain up to 75% pro-inflammatory fat, which is linked to multiple chronic illnesses. The American diet has around 20 times more inflammatory fat compared to anti-inflammatory fat, and it's this massive imbalance toward inflammation that leads to disease and weight gain.[11] If you don't remember or if you're reading the chapters out of order, inflammation is linked to chronic diseases like obesity, cardiovascular disease, Alzheimer's and type II diabetes.

Some industrial seed oils include:[12]

- All vegetable oils
- Safflower - 75% inflammatory fat (omega-6) and zero anti-inflammatory fat (omega-3)
- Sunflower - 65% inflammatory fat (omega-6) and zero anti-inflammatory fat (omega-3)
- Corn - 54% inflammatory fat (omega-6) and zero anti-inflammatory fat (omega-3)

- Cottonseed - 50% inflammatory fat (omega-6) and zero anti-inflammatory fat (omega-3)
- Sesame - 42% inflammatory fat (omega-6) and zero anti-inflammatory fat (omega-3)
- Peanut - 32% inflammatory fat (omega-6) and zero anti-inflammatory fat (omega-3)
- Soybean - 51% inflammatory fat (omega-6) and 7% anti-inflammatory fat (omega-3)

They are most prevalent in:

- Store-bought dressings
- Chips
- Crackers
- Restaurant food

HERE'S YOUR "RATIO" IF YOU MUST

I can try to tell you an exact ratio of proteins, healthy fats and carbohydrates that you should consume each day to attain the perfect body, but the truth is that everyone has different needs. What I know for sure is that the quality of the food you consume is top priority when it comes to what you should be putting on your plate. As the day progresses, your starchy carb intake should diminish and the overall size of your meals should be getting smaller. So, stick to a lot of vegetables, which will help maintain fullness while consuming fewer calories.

Check out the chart below for a very general ratio. Now in this program, you will be given the flexibility to exchange and substitute foods to your liking. I wouldn't stray very far from that ratio, but like I said, each person is different, so find out what works for you. And always keep in mind that QUALITY is always more important than ratio!

TYPE	PROTEIN	FAT	CARBOHYDRATES
ACTIVE INDIVIDUAL	25%	35%	40%
TROUBLE LOSING WEIGHT	30%	40%	30%

Remember, the goal of this program is to give you lifetime results. Will we really stick with the type of program that requires us to eat the exact same foods every day for the rest of our lives? No! Mixing up your lean proteins, vegetables and fruit choices will not only motivate you to stay on track with the program, but it can also be a lot of fun while providing a greater variety of nutrients. Trying a fruit that you never even knew existed could become your new favorite. Eating spaghetti squash instead of normal pasta cannot only benefit your waist line, but the rest of your body will also thank you for the extra nutrients you are putting into it. So branch out of your comfort zone a little and experiment with your journey toward total wellness by mixing up your meals.

*The Rant: When looking at macronutrients, you NEED to know that vegetables are going to remain crucial in your diet along with healthy fats and small amounts of quality proteins.

Lifestyle Scale	DESCRIPTION
Serving Size 1 Person Makes 1 Lifetime Result	**Difficulty** – Kicking addiction is never easy.
Grade Per Person	
Grade	**Time to Implement** – It takes 21 days to **create** or **replace** a habit.
Grade*	
Difficulty 9	**Importance** – If the **addiction** is not kicked, these foods are known to cause a number of otherwise **preventable** diseases.
Time to Implement 21 Days	
Importance 8	
*Amount is based off of the average person. Your personal results may be higher or lower depending on your specific needs.	

4

How to kick your food addiction

WHY ARE YOU ADDICTED?

First things first, you aren't alone when it comes to being addicted to food. There's a reason why Lays, the huge potato chip company, used the slogan, "Bet you can't eat just one!" The food industry has scientists working around the clock looking to expose what your body craves in order to create a product that will keep you coming back for more. However, the secret to outsmarting the food industry is simpler than you might ever think.

NATURE'S INTENTIONS ARE HONEST

Our bodies crave the big three when it comes to food – salt, sugar and fat. This is a built-in method that stems from our instincts to survive in nature.

Dating back to our ancestors, we have been able to detect which foods are safe in nature by how they taste.

*Sweet = safe
*Fatty = energy-rich
*Salty = preserves fluids
*Bitter = poison

When you ingest sugar and fat, you increase the amount of opiates being released into your brain. These opiates stimulate your brain to release dopamine (the "feel good hormone"), which gives you pleasure, alertness, concentration, euphoria and motivation.

FOOD INDUSTRY'S INTENTIONS ARE NOT

The food industry has been able to create "food-like products" with concentrated addictive tastes, all without having any nutritional value. Remember, it's their **job** to make you eat more of their company's food, whether it's healthy or not. These concentrated tastes overstimulate your taste buds in such a short period of time that your brain doesn't even have time to register how much you have actually ingested. It is concentrating on releasing the opiates, dopamine and that pleasurable feeling it has been looking for.

Typically, the food industry will eliminate the food's dietary fiber, dehydrate it, and then process it at extremely high temperatures (which strip its nutrients). If you took a cup of grapes and dehydrated them, you will be left with a quarter-cup of dried grapes (raisins), and then if you added sugar, artificial sweeteners and chocolate, now you have chocolate covered raisins. If you had to eat 1,000 calories worth of fresh grapes, you probably physically couldn't do it, BUT it's fairly easy to eat 1,000 calories worth of chocolate covered raisins.

Another example of the food industry's processing techniques is when they take out the fiber in brown rice, making it white rice. This not only completely changes the texture and flavor of the rice, but it also concentrates the sugar – and as we know, a concentration in sugar is never healthy for the body.

Addictive foods tend to be housed in packages in order to look tasty, convenient and attractive to consumers. Try to look for unpackaged foods, usually found on the perimeter of grocery stores, to avoid these processed foods and food-like products.

*Unfortunately, we as a society have not demonized the food industry like we have done with the tobacco industry, but isn't it really the same thing? They're both causing disease to spread like wild-fire throughout the world.

*A Connecticut College study of rats showed that Oreo filling, morphine and cocaine stimulated the pleasure portion of the brain. However, when rats were given the choice between the three, they chose the Oreo filling!

FOODS WITH A "PARACHUTE"

I like to use the example of a "parachute" when referring to addictive vs. whole foods. Foods with a "parachute" (whole foods) slowly digest, assimilate and absorb into your body at a rate in which you can fully receive all of the food's nutrients. Additionally, your body is going to be aware of how much of these foods it has ingested. Foods with no "parachute" (food-like products, processed foods) immediately digest, spike your blood sugar, cause chronic high insulin levels and typically provide you with little to no nutrients. Think of it like this: every time you eat, it's like you're jumping out of a plane at 10,000 feet (3,048 meters). Obviously, you would want to jump with a parachute, which can safely control your fall and guide you to the ground nice and easy. However, if you jump with no parachute, there's just the free-fall.

SUGAR ADDICTION: IT'S REAL

Sugar addiction isn't a surprising phenomenon considering that studies have shown it to be more addicting than drugs like cocaine and that over 80% of the foods found in grocery stores contain added sugars.[2, 3] From candy, soda and even hamburger meat, sugar is added to almost everything people ingest. And a high amount of sugar in your bloodstream can cause major damage to your body such as:

- Mineral depletion
- Immune repression
- Blood sugar imbalances
- Low brain function
- Increased cholesterol
- Heart disease
- Yeast overgrowth
- Poor teeth

Sugar depletes essential nutrients in your body like magnesium and B vitamins, which your body needs to convert tryptophan, an amino acid, to serotonin (the "happy hormone").

BE SUGAR SAVVY

You should understand which foods contain sugar, and which kinds of sugar at that. Make an inventory of higher sugar impact foods that you are currently consuming. Read the Nutrition Labels and Ingredient Lists on the back of packages to see how much sugar these foods actually have in them, and what quality of sugar. If any type of sugar is one of the three main ingredients in the package, PUT IT DOWN! Otherwise, take note of how many grams of sugar are in the package, the serving size and amount of servings that the package contains.

*Refer to Appendix (B) to learn about "How Do Sweeteners Rank?"

Making a journal of how much sugar you consume at each meal for even 3-5 days will help you identify foods you might be addicted to. So look at what you eat, at what time you eat and how you feel after you eat each food.

OWNING IT BY UNDERSTANDNING IT

The most important part of kicking your food addiction is to take responsibility for your addiction. You must fight back by lowering your addictive food intake slowly. Going cold turkey will only leave you feeling deprived, which will tempt you to revert back to your old ways. You have to tell yourself that you are choosing not to eat these addictive foods because you know that you will gain more compared to what you are giving up. This will put you in the right **mindset** to change your lifestyle for good!

Unconsciously, the body craves certain foods to heal itself with nutrients and to mask its pain with pleasure. This is why your body tells you to keep eating when you ingest foods with no nutrients like most addictive foods. It is attempting to gain nutrients from the food, but when they don't provide you with any (in processed and food-like products), your mind will keep telling you to eat until it is **nutritionally** satisfied. People confuse this unconscious reaction for a lack of willpower.

You should always look out for sugary, salty and fatty comfort foods. Ask yourself, are you eating this just to seek pleasure, or are you eating this for sustenance? When in doubt, find something that you love to do, like walking, watching TV, socializing, searching the web or exercising, and use that as your pleasure in place of addictive food.

*Satisfied vs. Stuffed – it takes your brain 20-30 minutes to catch up to your stomach. Think about foods without a "parachute" like a Twinkie - how many Twinkies can you eat in 20-30 minutes? I know I can eat too many!

A major problem with letting your emotions control your food intake is that when you receive the temporary pleasure to distract yourself from the emotion, once the pleasure goes away, the body will only be left with more pain. This starts a vicious cycle that will hardwire your brain to always seek more pleasure with poor food choices in an attempt to cover up pain.

It's never easy doing something like this alone. If you really want to make sure that you kick this addiction for good, do it with a friend, spouse or a colleague from work. The extra motivation from a teammate can give you the push you need to accomplish your ultimate goal.

FOCUS ON FIBER, FAT AND PROTEIN

You should focus on ingesting foods that are high in fiber (flaxseed, vegetables, small amounts of fruit), healthy fat (nuts, ghee, avocado) and small amounts of lean protein (grass-fed and hormone-free meats like chicken and turkey) too. Utilizing fiber, fat and protein will slow the digestion process, stabilize your blood sugar, help with satiety and increase your energy. You should **always** accompany each meal with vegetables since these will provide you with vitamins, minerals and fiber to keep you healthy and full!

*Satiety – a full sensation after a meal

*Some foods actually have fiber, fat **and** protein in them, like avocados, seeds and nuts!

You can swap out addictive food for almonds, avocados, bananas, lima beans, pumpkin seeds and sesame seeds as these other foods produce an increased level of dopamine as well. If you are craving sweets specifically, try podded peas, carrots, sweet potatoes, beets or rutabagas instead. These healthy alternatives are easy if you need to snack on something later in the night.

MAKE IT PERSONAL

Do you want to look better? Feel better? Avoid cancer, diabetes, stroke or heart disease? Setting a goal for yourself will help you reach tangible results in both the short- and long-run.

Like I said before, going cold turkey is a losing battle. Start by making shifts in your diet like using complex carbs in place of simple carbs. You'll find greater success by tapering down your usual unhealthy foods and by making better choices as the day goes on.

*The Rant: Once you understand that food addiction is not entirely your fault, you must create awareness around the problem in order to FIX it.

Lifestyle Scale	DESCRIPTION
Serving Size 1 Person Makes 1 Lifetime Result	
Grade Per Person	**Difficulty** – Changing your current habits by introducing **better** choices will not be difficult.
Grade	
Grade*	
Difficulty 3	**Time to Implement** – It takes 7 days to **start** making **better** choices.
Time to Implement 7 Days	**Importance** – Even if you can't make the **best** choices all the time, making **better** choices will lead you to success little by little.
Importance 6	
*Amount is based off of the average person. Your personal results may be higher or lower depending on your specific needs.	

5

Making better choices

When it comes to proper nutrition that leads to lasting results, it's about making BETTER choices. Now, when I say "better choices," I am NOT referring to "low fat" and "reduced fat" meal replacement products or processed foods. Typically, these foods are really just replacing the fat with a high amount of sugar, and if you don't know by now, sugar is what is essentially making us fat! Additionally, when I say to start eating breakfast, this doesn't mean eating cereal or a bagel with cream cheese, because neither are healthy, nor will they increase your metabolism.

Making better choices means that you need to eat foods that are coming from Mother Nature, not major manufacturers. Each time you reach for food, make the **better** choice compared to what you did when you started. Every time you pick up anything that is harmful say, "I'm not going to eat this because I'm going to gain way more than I will give up." I would love to be able to tell you the best choices out there and have you go to the market and buy exactly what I say, but I know that isn't a reality. Everyone has their different food preferences that lead them down their unique paths. This does NOT mean that those paths don't still end up at total wellness, but one person's path might take a little longer compared to another. With consistency, we will all get there in due time, friends!

FOODS AGE JUST LIKE US

Foods lose their nutritional value with age, so finding fresh foods to eat is important. If you take a look at iceberg lettuce from the grocery store, it has about the same nutritional value as a piece of paper. If you take a look at some greens grown right around the corner from a local farmer, these are filled with dense nutrients, vitamins and ENERGY! So, what I am really trying to say is to skip the long, drawn-out process that is involved when purchasing foods from a store, which causes your food to lose its nutritional value. Instead, go to a farmer's market – not only is the food going to taste much better but it also supports your local economy.

You should also be eating seasonally. There's a season for every fruit, vegetable and even some meats. You can look these details up easily on-line or by checking with a local farmer, but if you can still get strawberries in the grocery store in mid-December, for example, that isn't right. Not only are you MONTHS removed from strawberry season, but the amount of preservatives put into that fruit to make it last that long is as ridiculous as it is unhealthy, and it could have been harvested way before it was ripe and placed in cold storage, where it more rapidly loses its nutritional value.

WHAT'S WITH ORGANIC?

There is a huge community out there, mostly the healthy population, that swears by organic food products, but there are others, mostly the big farming population, that claim "organic" doesn't matter. So does "organic" really matter? The simplest way to say it is YES!

Organic is really telling the consumer that the products they are buying are being protected by the U.S. Department of Agriculture (USDA) to make sure certain unhealthy, synthetic and non-synthetic substances are not being used while farms are producing their food. You are probably thinking to yourself, "Isn't that how food is produced anyway?" The sad truth is that unfortunately it's not, and someone has to fight for it to come to you as clean as possible.

According to the Organic Consumers Association (OCA), organic foods are not allowed to contain or be produced with: [1]

- Food additives
- Flavor enhancers like MSG
- Artificial sweeteners such as aspartame and high-fructose corn syrup
- Contaminants like mercury
- Preservatives like sodium nitrate
- Pesticides
- Genetically Modified (GMO) crops
- Antibiotics
- Growth hormones
- Arsenic
- Byproducts of corn ethanol production
- Toxic sewage sludge
- Sewage water
- Coal waste

If you didn't catch a couple of those, yes, I said sewage sludge, growth hormones and pesticides. You would think that anything classified as "food" shouldn't be produced with ANYTHING listed above, but the harsh reality is that most of our "food" is. This is why looking for a product labeled with the "USDA Organic" seal is EXTREMELY important.

IT'S WORTH IT

Now, when people think organic, they often automatically think, "ORGANIC! That's so expensive!" Well, the cost is justified through the benefits that you are going to receive from the food itself. **Even though, according to the OCA, organic foods are roughly 20% more expensive than non-organic, on average, organic foods are going to provide you with 25% MORE vitamins and minerals compared to the latter.**[1] If you aren't worried about the toxic sewage sludge, maybe this will convince you to purchase a higher quality food like organic products.

The bottom line is that when you are choosing organic foods, your body will be able to lose fat more rapidly because you are ingesting less toxic loads from horrible foods, and fewer toxins means faster fat loss. The reason being is that your body is only able to handle so many toxins at one time, and most likely, it already has a massive storage of toxins within your fat cells. Furthermore, the majorities of overweight people have nutrient deficiencies, so the increased amount of nutrients found in organic foods will help address the deficiency!

These recommendations will help you to make positive changes in your diet by consuming QUALITY foods compared to food-like substances. Making a single better choice leads to another, which leads to one more and so on. The next thing you know, those better choices each day end up leading you to your ultimate goal without you even noticing it! Think before you act, and always ask yourself, "How will this decision affect how I feel afterward?" Not only do these healthy choices taste better, but they will make a huge difference in your diet.

THE "DIRTY DOZEN PLUS" & "CLEAN FIFTEEN"

Every year, the Environmental Working Group (EWG) gives a list of foods that are at the highest risk for pesticides in your diet.[2] These are the foods that you should always try to choose as organic. Since I am telling you the truth about this world, only SOME of your foods are more important when it comes to choosing organic, which means that your entire grocery cart doesn't have to be organic. Please visit www.ewg.org for the current shopper's guide to pesticides in produce.

CAN I AFFORD TO EAT LIKE THIS?

At first glance, some of the healthy food options might look expensive, but always keep in mind that this is a FAT LOSS program, so you will be eating less. If you are saying to yourself, "I have no clue how to make any of these foods. What am I going to do?" Don't worry about it! Day by day, you will start becoming a better and healthier chef, which will result in saving money by eating out less often, but still enjoying a delicious and nutritious meal. When you choose quality ingredients, your body will **naturally** be less hungry because it will sense that it is receiving a substantial amount of nutrients that it needs to properly function. On the flip side, most processed foods contain genetically altered, pro-inflammatory macronutrients, too much salt, sugar, unhealthy food additives, pesticides and hormones. Each of these items, but especially a combination of them, contributes to a lack of the essential nutrients causing your metabolism to slow and your hunger to increase.

I know how tough finances can be. A lot of people tell me that they don't have enough money to eat healthy, but what they are doing incorrectly is looking for the wrong type of food at the wrong time of the year. Like I said before, you have to learn how to eat seasonally because even though you can get asparagus in the middle of January, they aren't fresh, and they're most likely more expensive compared to getting them in July. A good tip to help you save some money is to stock up on healthy food when it's on sale. The freezer can become your best friend when you buy food in bulk. Just remember that the longer you keep your food frozen, the more nutrients that will be lost. If preparation time is becoming an issue and you want to save some time at the grocery store, use fresh fruits and vegetables at the beginning of the week, then switch to frozen toward the end of the week. Whatever you have for dinner can always become tomorrow's lunch. You can also use a leftover protein like chicken or turkey for a salad or soup the next day.

BETTER CHOICES CHECKLIST

- Trade in your normal bread for gluten-free brands like "Food for Life," which include Bhutanese red rice, brown rice, exotic black rice, rice pecan, rice almond and rice millet breads. Any of the "Ezekiel" breads are also okay, but they do have some gluten in them, so it's not an ideal choice, but it is a **better** choice.
- Mashed cauliflower can replace your mashed potatoes.
- Brown, black or red rice can substitute for white rice.
- Organic salsa can be used in place of ketchup.
- Swap out white potatoes in exchange for red potatoes, yams or sweet potatoes.
- Replace normal dairy yogurt with cultured almond milk yogurt or cultured coconut milk yogurt. Just make sure that they have less than 15 grams of sugar per serving.
- Eliminate white pasta and replace it with rice or quinoa pasta or, better yet, spaghetti squash.
- If you NEED to have a tortilla, find a brown rice version.
- If you are consuming any chocolate on occasion, use organic 85% or over dark chocolate.

ELIMINATE LIQUID EMPTY CALORIES TO ACCELERATE FAT LOSS

- Any sweetened teas should be replaced with unsweetened green tea, black tea or any organic tea of choice.

- Replace juice and soda with carbonated water. To give it a little more flavor, add lemon or lime slices.
- Eliminate all coffee creamers, both low-fat and no fat. Replace it with unsweetened almond or coconut milk creamers. Make sure that you are drinking them near your meal times in order to accelerate fat loss in between ingesting calories.
- Remove all sugar from your meals and beverages! If you need a natural sweetener, use small amounts of xylitol or stevia in its place.
- Any juices should be replaced with their entire form of the fruit. For example, orange juice should be replaced by consuming a whole orange. It sounds like it wouldn't make a difference, but the amount of fiber that you consume from the whole fruit helps with keeping your metabolism elevated and helps to remove toxins from the body.
- Because so much of the corn we see today is genetically modified (GMO), remove it completely from your diet and replace it with presoaked beans. Corn is also extremely high in sugar, which doesn't do you any favors.
- Lose the light olive oil and replace it with cold-pressed extra-virgin olive oil. First press cold-pressed extra virgin olive oil is the best.
- Eliminate ALL animal milk from your diet! Instead, try almond milk, coconut milk, hemp milk or rice milk.
- Eliminate all cheese products and replace them with non-dairy cheese or other non-soy alternatives.

TREATS FOR EVERY NOW AND AGAIN

- Try "So Delicious" no sugar added coconut milk (or almond milk) dairy-free ice cream. It comes in several flavors, which are all delicious, including butter pecan, cherry amaretto, chocolate, vanilla, cookies & cream, mint chip, chocolate brownie almond, gluten-free cookie dough and more!

- Try some frozen banana with almond butter "ice cream" for a change-up! Just freeze peeled one-inch banana chunks overnight. Take enough chunks that would amount to one full banana and put it in a blender with 2 tablespoons of almond butter. Blend until it reaches an ice cream-like texture and enjoy!

WORRIED ABOUT CALCIUM? DITCH THE DAIRY

- Dark green, leafy veggies are really the best.
- Some others include almonds, bok choy, broccoli, nopals, cauliflower, collard greens, cucumbers, dates, figs, kale, oranges, romaine lettuce, sea vegetables, sesame seeds, spinach, sunflower seeds, turnip greens and watercress.

NEED A SALAD DRESSING?

Apple Cider Vinaigrette
1 cup raw apple cider vinegar
2 tablespoons seeded Dijon mustard
¾ cup cold-pressed extra-virgin olive oil
Juice from half of a lemon
½ cup finely chopped fresh chives
½ tablespoon of curry powder

Blend all the ingredients together in your blender until they are well distributed. This dressing is **highly recommended** for any salads. The apple cider vinegar will help to increase the healthy gut bacteria in your gastrointestinal tract.

*The Rant: Once you are able to string along a bunch of little healthy choices daily, weekly and then monthly, you will be surprised what those choices can add up to in a year from now!

Lifestyle Scale	DESCRIPTION
Serving Size 1 Person Makes 1 Lifetime Result	**Difficulty** – Once you start using fat for energy, it is fairly difficult to push through the side effects of detoxifying your body.
Grade Per Person	
Grade	
Grade*	
Difficulty 5	**Time to Implement** – It takes around 3 days to **deplete** your carb storage before you can **access** fat deposits.
Time to Implement 3 Days	**Importance** – This is **crucial** information when trying to lose **strictly** body fat.
Importance 8	
*Amount is based off of the average person. Your personal results may be higher or lower depending on your specific needs.	

6

Positioning fat loss

Positioning fat loss is the ability to increase your metabolism to a point where you are constantly burning fat. Unfortunately, it's not a process that happens overnight – it's something that you have to stick to for a while in order to see real results.

YOUR ENERGY BANKS

A way that you can look at your fat loss is to think of glycogen storage in your muscles and liver as "energy banks." As long as you have these energy banks, your brain will not need to take out a loan from your fat cells. So, if you can lower the amount of stored energy in these energy banks, you can burn more fat cells. How do you do this? Well, by incorporating all the wellness tips you are learning collectively, which will help this to happen easier and more naturally.

> * Glycogen storage: Stored energy in your muscles and liver, roughly 75% water 25% carbohydrates.

To make a huge dent in these energy banks, you can exercise and lower your total amount of calories that you ingest during the day. When you do this, you are lowering the amount of stored energy in these banks, which allows fat to be used as energy. However, make sure that it's **strategic** and NOT to a point where you are starving yourself.

The body follows the path of least resistance, so it will first burn through the calories that you ingest, then to the stored energy banks in your liver and muscles. The energy pulled from your liver is meant to stabilize your blood-sugar level, and the energy pulled from your muscles is used to fuel activity. Once these banks are depleted of their carbohydrate reserves, your body will then break down body fat for energy. The system works more efficiently when you eat healthy foods because your body does not have to spend any energy detoxifying the food that you ingest, and it will be provided with the nutrients that it needs in order to increase your metabolism.

IN THIS CASE: SMALLER IS BETTER

When you eat smaller meals (I recommend 4-6 small, unprocessed, healthy meals each day), they will be burned off quickly so that your body can easily dip into your fat stores, which allows you to use more of your fat-burning hormones like glucagon. This is just one hormone signaling the release of stored fat cells to be used as energy, which increases your available energy and decreases your hunger!

When you start utilizing more fat as energy, you might initially become hungry, fatigued, moody, have low blood sugar and/or experience a slight headache. The amount and intensity of these temporary side effects depends largely on how many toxins are stored in your fat cells from the food that was turned into the fat originally. Either way, your body will adapt within a few days, and then you will feel better than ever!

FIGHT THE URGE TO BINGE

You should be eating more in the morning as this will set you up for the whole day with vitamins, minerals, energy and information. You might not need to eat all five meals on any given day. It could be four or it could be six depending on your schedule and activity level. Furthermore, your spacing doesn't always have to be three hours, but what I have seen is that waiting over four hours tends to lead to poor choices and binge eating. The last thing that you want after working so hard is to start over following a binge meal.

Binge eating, which is common when dieters do not eat enough quality foods during the day, leads to fat storage because it allows extra energy to float in your blood stream with no place to go. Spacing out your meals and snacks will, in reality, benefit you in the long run. The key to success is to have portion control when it comes to each of your meals. They should be divided up into three meals per day like breakfast, lunch and dinner; then two or three small snacks made up of a quality, plant-based fiber like veggies, a lean protein and healthy fat.

The general recommendation for fat loss is five meals a day. If you eat too many meals, you won't give your body enough time to utilize fat in between, but if you eat too little, it can lower your metabolism and increase your risk of binging.

*Many people tend to eat perfectly for 3 to 5 days, but fall off the edge on the weekends – this will put you back to square one. You MUST know that eating clean for an extended period of time will give you accelerated results.

NO MORE "NIBBLING"

Remember, anything that you ingest will have to be digested and absorbed by your body. This means ANY food you consume, whether a whole meal or just a nibble, counts toward your total daily calories. Even chewing "sugar-free" gums, which contain horrible artificial sweeteners, will cause your body to secrete insulin. This means your body will NOT be secreting your fat-burning hormones, like glucagon. No glucagon = no fat loss! So, ANYTHING you put in your mouth has to be utilized. Therefore, it's **extremely** important that you never eat anything in between meals. A nibble here and there DOES make a difference when it comes to fat loss. Let your body become used to using its own fat for energy and you will be on your way to major results!

*The Rant: Timing does matter when it comes to burning strictly fat — fighting the urge to eat in between meals will **supercharge** your fat loss.

Lifestyle Scale	DESCRIPTION
Serving Size 1 Person Makes 1 Lifetime Result	**Difficulty** – It is hard to break a **habit**, especially if that food is a **favorite**.
Grade Per Person	
Grade	
Grade*	**Time to Implement** – It takes 30 days to identify the **exact** food allergen.
Difficulty 6	
Time to Implement 30 Days	**Importance** – If allergic, this can allow you to make **huge** strides in your fitness goals.
Importance 5	
*Amount is based off of the average person. Your personal results may be higher or lower depending on your specific needs.	

7

Eliminate gluten & dairy

E liminating two of the most common food allergens – gluten and dairy – will shape up your diet for success whether you're allergic to them or not!

Gluten and dairy are the top food proteins that lead to intolerance, which may cause inflammation and inhibit your body's natural ability to reduce fat. Removing both is a lot easier than you might have thought, and doing so is not only a great way to start your wellness journey, but it will set you up for the best chance at success.

*Intolerance – rejection of the food protein leading to a variety of side effects including acne, inflammation, bloating, gas, weight gain, etc.

If dairy is the only way you like to get protein, and especially if you ingest dairy with every meal, eliminating and replacing it with alternatives will reduce inflammation even if you're not allergic.[1,2] If, after cutting out dairy from your diet, you experience fat loss, reduced bloating, less gas and decreased anthropomorphic measurements (bodyweight & waist-to-hip ratio), it would be correct to assume that this course of action was a positive choice and should be maintained.

The other common allergy is to gluten, or what is known as Celiac disease.[3] Whether you have a full-blown allergy or just a slight sensitivity, deleting gluten from your diet is beneficial. Celiac is triggered by the protein, gluten, which is found in barley, wheat, rye and spelt. Celiac disease is on the rise, which can be complicated by the synergistic effect of several environmental prompts.

*Environmental prompts: Foods are prepared differently than they were in the past and the introduction of genetically modified foods in our food supplies has affected the quality of our food.

There are other food-based allergens that may be negatively impacting your wellness, and an elimination diet is a useful tactic in determining a food sensitivity or allergy. The method works by removing all of your suspect foods from your diet for one month, then adding these foods back into your diet **slowly** and **one at a time**. If you are trying to figure out an allergen, introduce the problematic food for an entire day and wait two days without eating that or other foods you suspect cause irritability. If symptoms appear within two days, including looking and feeling worse, assume that you've found an allergen! If this food doesn't cause symptoms, wait to add it back into your diet until you've tested ALL suspected foods.

* Whey protein isolate sweetened with stevia and grass-fed organic ghee are better tolerated by the body and can be used during the elimination diet.

DAIRY

Eliminate all dairy products, including*:

- Milk
- Cream
- Cheese
- Cottage cheese
- Yogurt
- Butter
- Ice cream
- Frozen yogurt
- Hidden dairy
- Caramel candy
- Carob candies
- Casein
- Caseinates
- Custard
- Curds
- Lactalbumin
- Goat's milk
- Milk chocolate
- Nougat
- Protein hydrolysate
- Semisweet chocolate
- Pudding
- Whey
- Brown sugar flavoring
- Butter flavoring
- Caramel flavoring
- Coconut cream flavoring
- "Natural flavoring"
- Simplesse

* There are several dairy substitutes on the market like nut alternatives and coconut products. However, make sure to avoid all soy products due to their high level of processing.

GLUTEN

Gluten-free products have not been proven to be better than the normal versions of those products. I know. But gluten has been shown to cause inflammation within a large majority of the population, and chronic inflammation leads to weight gain in the long run. So when I say gluten-free, I don't want you to choose garbage food-like products like cookies and other desserts that are gluten-free. The rules still apply here: choose **quality, real** food ONLY!

When I say for you to eliminate gluten, avoid any foods that contain*:

- Wheat
- Spelt
- Kamut
- Rye
- Barley
- Malt
- Atta
- Bal ahar
- Bread flour
- Bulgar
- Cake flour
- Cereal extract
- Couscous
- Cracked wheat
- Durum flour
- Farina
- Graham flour
- High-gluten flour
- High-protein flour
- Kamut flour
- Laubina
- Leche alim
- Malted cereals
- Minchin
- Multi-grain products
- Puffed wheat
- Red wheat flakes
- Rolled wheat
- Semolina
- Shredded wheat
- Soft wheat flour
- Spelt
- Superamine
- Triticale

- Vital gluten
- Vitalia macaroni
- Wheat protein powder
- Wheat starch
- Wheat tempeh
- White flour
- Whole-wheat berries

- Gelatinized starch
- Hydrolyzed vegetable protein
- Modified food starch
- Starch
- Vegetable gum
- Vegetable starch

Substitute these with*:

- Brown rice
- Millet
- Buckwheat
- Quinoa
- Gluten-free flour products
- Potatoes
- Arrowroot products

*Notes from UW Integrative Medicine[4]

*The Rant: Even if you aren't allergic to dairy or gluten, eliminating these two types of foods will increase your body's ability to burn fat.

Lifestyle Scale	DESCRIPTION
Serving Size 1 Person Makes 1 Lifetime Result	**Difficulty** – Choosing the **right** foods in order to help your digestive tract will **not** be very difficult.
Grade Per Person	
Grade	
Grade*	
Difficulty 4	**Time to Implement** – It takes 21 days to **create** or **replace** a habit.
Time to Implement 21 Days	**Importance** – **Understanding** this and **implementing** these tips will make massive progress.
Importance 5	
*Amount is based off of the average person. Your personal results may be higher or lower depending on your specific needs.	

8

A healthy gut = increased fat loss

Let's go back to the basics because it's the little things that add up to the big results!

Did you ever have a gut feeling? The gut has way more intelligence than we may ever fully understand. Your gastrointestinal (GI) tract constantly communicates with your immune system, brain and **fat cells**! If you are sick, tired and having trouble losing weight, improving your gut health may be the missing link!

So, what exactly is your GI tract? It's a hollow tube that separates your body from the outside world, which extends from your mouth to your anus. It's about 25 to 30 feet long, and its surface area is equivalent to the size of a tennis court! The GI's functions include digesting nutrients, absorbing nutrients, keeping out non-nutrients and identifying the body's "friends" and "foes." Understanding how this system works, and then how to heal it, will be critical for permanent fat loss.

HEALTH STARTS IN YOUR GUT

Except for oxygen, everything your body needs has to be processed and absorbed in your gut. Statistics show that approximately 60-80% of your immune system is found in the gastrointestinal tract, and nearly 90% of serotonin, the happy hormone, is found there as well.

A research article was conducted by the National Academy of Science where they compared mice with healthy gut bacteria to mice with un-healthy gut bacteria[1,2]. The research revealed that the mice with the healthy digestive tract lost weight and had more energy! Think about it, without proper GI function, there is no health and your fat loss can be halted.

IT'S MORE THAN JUST DIGESTION

Repairing and maintaining the health of your GI tract is critical to increasing your metabolism. If you can somehow relax in this fast-paced world we live in, you can switch the body into what is called the parasympathetic nervous system (PNS). The parasympathetic nervous system and sympathetic nervous system are part of the autonomic nervous system. The autonomic nervous system works mainly on a conscious level that controls visceral functions like how you digest food, how rapidly your heart beats, how fast you breathe and your sexual arousal. The PNS is known as being the "rest and digest system," and the sympathetic nervous system is known as the "fight or flight response." You are going to want your body in the parasympathetic nervous system in order to calm your nerves prior to eating.

Marc David, author of *The Slow Down Diet*, explains that 40-60% of your digestion and energy burning starts in your brain.[3] What this really means is that your ability to assimilate, digest and burn calories come from the scientific impact of your thoughts. So your beliefs, stress, relations, pleasure, breathing and awareness can actually affect your digestion! Even the smell, satisfaction, pleasure, taste and the presentation of a meal can make a difference in how your body responds to the food.

POWER OF THE PNS

So how do you use the power of the parasympathetic nervous system in relation to digestive health? It's a two-step process: the first step, like everything else I talk about, is based on creating awareness. Say to yourself, "Okay, I am going to eat a meal. I need to simply relax, because if I relax I will increase my metabolism, and more so, eliminate any digestive issues." It sounds like some mumbo jumbo, but believe me, it works. Step two is taking 6 to 10 deep breaths prior to a meal. Some of my clients like to say a prayer or use meditation. Remember, it's what works for you that matters!

PIT STOPS

In order for your food to properly digest, it has to go through some major pit stops along the way through the GI tract. The first pit stop on its journey is your mouth. This is where you are going to be chewing your food thoroughly, and your salivary glands are going to release amylase (saliva) to assist in breaking down carbohydrates. Notice that I said to chew thoroughly! This should be more natural now that you're in the parasympathetic nervous system drive. Additionally, the more you chew your food, the easier it is going to be for your GI tract to absorb nutrients. However, keep in mind that the bigger the meal you ingest, the harder it is for your GI tract to digest it. When you eat smaller meals, the body is going to preserve its resources, which will help you to assimilate the nutrients more efficiently. Also, gas, bloating and other digestive problems will disappear.

Pit stop number two, which is your stomach, secretes hydrochloric acid, which destroys food-borne invaders such as bacteria and parasites. Your stomach also produces an enzyme called pepsin, which breaks down proteins. To increase your stomach acid naturally, squeeze half of a fresh lemon or a tablespoon of raw, fermented, unpasteurized apple cider vinegar into water, and drink it 20 minutes prior to eating your high-protein meals.

*Hydrochloric acid: a highly acidic juice formed in the stomach.

* If you take antacids, you are hindering the digestion of protein and introducing food borne pathogens into your intestines by decreasing the amount of hydrochloric acid in your stomach.

*Heartburn can be caused by **either** an overabundance or a lack of stomach acid!

Your food's third pit stop is the small intestines, which are nearly 20 feet long, and are divided into three distinct parts: the duodenum, the jejunum and the ilium. The duodenum releases pancreatic lipase enzymes and bile from the gallbladder to help the chemical breakdown of fats and carbohydrates. The jejunum, which is the largest, has specific abilities to absorb broken down carbohydrates and proteins. Lastly, the ilium acts as the cleanup station that absorbs residual vitamins, minerals and bile salts.

*Pancreatic lipase: Primary enzyme that breaks down dietary fat molecules in the human digestive system.

The large intestines (colon) are our final pit stop, which absorbs water and vitamins while converting digested foods into feces. While you have several bacteria throughout your digestive tract, you have a little in your mouth, nothing in your stomach, a few in your small intestines, and the highest concentration in your large intestines. Supplementing with probiotics and eating fermented foods are so critical because our gut has 100 trillion micro-organisms in it. Yes, 100 trillion. And problems occur if too many are bad bacteria. Antibiotic therapy, alcohol consumption, stress, non-steroidal anti-inflammatory drugs (NSAIDs) and the average

American diet, which is full of processed foods and sugar, all cause inflammation and give rise to the bad bacteria!

GOOD GUYS IN THE GUT

All the supplements in the world will not help if you eat poor quality food or a food that you have an allergy to. The food choices recommended on this program are anti-inflammatory and will be the first step in healing the gut. Fermented foods and a probiotic will help crowd out the bad bacteria. The good bacteria can help with irritable bowel syndrome (IBS) and inflammatory bowel disease (IBD), protect against infection by pathogens like yeast, decrease the side effects of antibiotic therapy and cortical steroids. The good bacteria also helps prevent leaky gut syndrome, which causes large proteins to enter the body that aren't supposed to, which leads to an all-out immune response that attaches to the protein, which is thought to be a cause of many auto-immune diseases.

HOW DO YOU REPAIR IT?

Recommendations on **how** to improve digestive health:

- Get into a relaxed state of mind prior to beginning each meal
- Really chew that food
- Never overeat
- Eliminate processed foods
- Increase dietary fiber from plant-based nutrition
- Limit water consumption **with** your meals (drink water 45 minutes prior to your meal)
- Take a probiotic
- Eat fermented foods
- Use 1 tablespoon of lemon juice or raw apple cider vinegar in water 20 minutes prior to meal (especially if it's a high protein meal)
- Exercise to help food move through your digestive tract
- Eat anti-inflammatory omega-3 fats and the foods recommended in this program

*RAW APPLE CIDER VINEGAR

- This is used to aid in optimal digestion while encouraging healthy bacterial growth in your gastrointestinal tract
- Sip 1 tablespoon of raw apple cider vinegar dissolved in a cup of water 20 minutes prior to your meal to aid in digestion
- The vinegar has to be **raw** and **unfiltered**
- You can also use it in your salad dressing when prompted to use vinegar

*The Rant: Your body's ability to burn fat will be hindered, especially in the long-run, without proper GI function. Your overall health will also suffer.

Lifestyle Scale	DESCRIPTION
Serving Size 1 Person Makes 1 Lifetime Result	**Difficulty** – For people who do not already do so, starting will be difficult **at first** but **easier** as it goes on.
Grade Per Person	
Grade	
Grade*	**Time to Implement** – It takes 21 days to **create** or **replace** a habit.
Difficulty 5	
Time to Implement 21 Days	**Importance** – Breakfast will set you up for your **entire day** with **crucial** energy.
Importance 7	
*Amount is based off of the average person. Your personal results may be higher or lower depending on your specific needs.	

9

Portion control is vital

Portions and servings are something that really mess up dieters, but understanding them is going to put you leaps and bounds ahead of where you were before. Many restaurants serve monstrous portions of what **could** have been a healthy meal. Entrees are often 2,000 calories, and of course you're going to feel like you should down the whole meal in one sitting. You might also feel the same way when eating at home, but just because you have the food made doesn't mean you should eat it all in one sitting. Making the clear distinction between a portion and a serving will help you gain massive ground in your program.

PORTIONS VS. SERVINGS

Well, what's the difference between the two? A "portion" is the amount of food that you choose to eat for a meal or snack during one sitting. A "serving" is a measured amount of food or drink but not necessarily how much you will be consuming. Checking nutrition labels shows that, more often than not, foods can come in a "one portion" box or package, but contain more than one serving! One of the worst offenders would be processed foods and sodas. A 20 oz. soda is usually consumed by one person in a single sitting, but there are actually 2.5 servings in that bottle and 65 grams of total sugar! The companies who make the soda know that the consumer is going to drink the entire bottle, but they don't want to admit to how much sugar is really in their beverage. Yes, it's a deceiving, conniving way to get people to buy a product, so please check the labels on your foods before you purchase them to avoid setting yourself back in your program.

WHAT ARE SERVING SIZES FOR DIFFERENT FOODS?

Some of the foods listed below are **unhealthy** and you shouldn't be eating them on this program. However, I'm using them to illustrate a point. If you insist, you can also measure and weigh all of your foods, which will let you see how large or small portions really are, but the process is time-consuming and energy draining. So to give you an idea on portions and servings, I recommend that you study the guidelines below, and practice measuring and weighing foods in all of the categories.

*Not a recommended food source

- Bread, cereal, rice and pasta
  - 1 slice of bread*
  - 1 small roll*
  - 5-6 crackers*
  - ½ cup rice, pasta or cooked cereal*

- Fruit
  - One medium-size fruit
  - 1 cup of berries
- Veggies
  - ½ cup no matter how prepared
  - 1 cup of leafy raw veggies like spinach
- Dairy
  - 1 cup of milk*
  - 2 ounces of cheese*
- Meat/Protein
  - 2-3 ounces
  - 1 egg
- Fats
  - 2 tablespoons of nut butter
  - 1 tablespoon of oil
  - 1 tablespoon of butter
  - 1 tablespoon of salad dressing

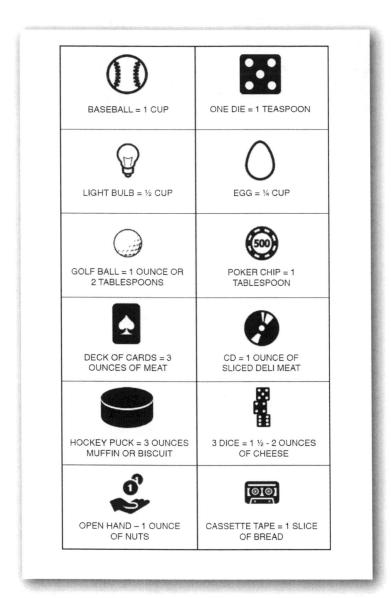

BASEBALL = 1 CUP	ONE DIE = 1 TEASPOON
LIGHT BULB = ½ CUP	EGG = ¼ CUP
GOLF BALL = 1 OUNCE OR 2 TABLESPOONS	POKER CHIP = 1 TABLESPOON
DECK OF CARDS = 3 OUNCES OF MEAT	CD = 1 OUNCE OF SLICED DELI MEAT
HOCKEY PUCK = 3 OUNCES MUFFIN OR BISCUIT	3 DICE = 1 ½ - 2 OUNCES OF CHEESE
OPEN HAND – 1 OUNCE OF NUTS	CASSETTE TAPE = 1 SLICE OF BREAD

*The Rant: When beginning the program, understanding how much you are ingesting will help you understand any possible struggles. If you are choosing quality foods, your body will automatically portion control itself because it is receiving more nutrients.

Lifestyle Scale	DESCRIPTION
Serving Size 1 Person Makes 1 Lifetime Result	**Difficulty** – Following this guideline will be **difficult** at first and **easy** as it goes on.
Grade Per Person	
Grade	
Grade*	**Time to Implement** – It is a **5-Day Breakdown**.
Difficulty 7	
Time to Implement 5 Days	**Importance** – Following this breakdown will give you an **idea** on the **program** as a whole.
Importance 7	
*Amount is based off of the average person. Your personal results may be higher or lower depending on your specific needs.	

10

Five-day breakdown

We all have days when we eat poorly because time is an issue. We choose fast foods, convenience foods and processed pastries instead of quality veggies, fruits, proteins and fats. But time is no longer an excuse with this program.

The meals provided below are an outline to show you how easy it is to get rid of processed foods in your life! The suggested foods compared to others will create the energy and information your body needs in order to sustain fat loss over the long-haul. Be sure to study the chapter "Macronutrients: The Comprehensive Breakdown," which goes over some quality guidelines about nutrition. The more **quality** foods you have, the **faster** your body will **burn fat,** and the better it will **preserve** its **muscle,** which is the number-one driver of your metabolism. So having more muscle means fat will be burned twenty-four hours a day!

As an example only, this is a **Five-Day Breakdown** of meals for both men and women. On the low-end, the calories for women are around 1,200 to 1,300, and men's calories are around 1,600 to 1,800. You may have to adjust this depending on a few variables.

The first variable is **age**. Normally the older we get, the fewer calories we can consume. Next is your **activity level**. If you are extremely active, you should increase your calories. If so, you have the flexibility to increase your healthy carbs and fats SLIGHTLY. The last variable is your **body mass index**. If you are on the higher end of the body mass index you also have the ability to increase your healthy carbs and fats SLIGHTLY. Nevertheless, remember if you're trying to lose weight, increasing your calorie intake too much will obviously slow your progress. You also want to be careful not to overestimate how many calories you're actually burning exercising at the gym, going for a short walk or playing volleyball at a family barbeque. All that activity might only burn 100-200 calories every day, which is roughly equivalent to burning off one snack as outlined below.

SCENARIO

Say you and your significant other are following this program using the supplemental meals. The two of you are eating the same meals each day, which are made with **real food**, and let's pretend that you have identical food preferences. You can make your meals larger (perfect for men) or smaller (perfect for women) by adjusting the serving. The theory and time saving techniques are exactly alike, so the only major difference is determined by the serving size, so pay attention.

*All of the following recipes can be found at
www.ItsFatLossNotWeightLoss.com along with the newest version of my
Five-Day Breakdown.

DAY 1

Breakfast
Women: JK Breakfast Omelet (1 serving)
Total Meal Calories: 349.91
Men: JK Breakfast Omelet (1 serving) + Fresh Strawberries (2 cups whole)
Total Meal Calories: 443.91

Snack 1
Women: JK Orange with Walnuts (1 serving)
Total Meal Calories: 153.56
Men: JK Orange with Walnuts (1 serving) + JK Mixed Nuts (1/2 serving)
Total Meal Calories: 264.26

Lunch
Women: JK Greek Quinoa Salad (1 serving)
Total Meal Calories: 290.41
Men: JK Greek Quinoa Salad (1.5 servings)
Total Meal Calories: 435.61

Snack 2
Women: JK Apple Slices with Almond Butter (1 serving)
Total Meal Calories: 200.00
Men: JK Apple Slices with Almond Butter (1 serving)
Total Meal Calories: 200.00

Dinner
Women: JK Broiled Paprika and Lime Chicken with Quinoa and Broccoli (3/4 serving)
Total Meal Calories: 264.35
Men: JK Broiled Paprika and Lime Chicken with Quinoa and Broccoli (1 serving)
Total Meal Calories: 352.47

Women Total Calories per Day: 1,258.23

Men Total Calories per Day: 1,696.25

EXPLANATION

By making three servings of the Breakfast Omelet, you can store the leftovers in the refrigerator inside an airtight glass container for quick reheating. This will allow you to have one serving each morning for three consecutive days. Talk about a time saver! Next, pack two fast and easy snacks that are completely interchangeable. If you have a desk drawer, you can bring most of them to work with you and put the cold items in a cooler or the company's refrigerator. Now all you have to worry about is dinner.

*A glass container will protect your food from toxic chemicals found in plastic containers.

DAY 2

Breakfast
Women: JK Breakfast Omelet (1 serving)
Total Meal Calories: 349.91
Men: JK Breakfast Omelet (1 serving) + Pear – medium with peel (1 whole)
Total Meal Calories: 447.91

Snack 1
Women: JK Grapes with Cashews (1 serving)
Total Meal Calories: 143.32
Men: JK Grapes with Cashews (1.5 servings)
Total Meal Calories: 214.98

Lunch
Women: JK Broiled Paprika and Lime Chicken with Quinoa and Broccoli (1 serving)
Total Meal Calories: 352.47

Men: JK Broiled Paprika and Lime Chicken with Quinoa and Broccoli (1.5 servings)
Total Meal Calories: 528.70

Snack 2
Women: JK Carrots with Hummus (1 serving)
Total Meal Calories: 129.73
Men: JK Carrots with Hummus (1.5 servings)
Total Meal Calories: 194.59

Dinner
Women: JK Haddock with Kale and (optional) Brown Rice (1 serving)
Total Meal Calories: 278.45
Men: JK Haddock with Kale and (optional) Brown Rice (1 serving)
Total Meal Calories: 278.45

Women Total Calories per Day: 1,253.88

Men Total Calories per Day: 1,664.73

EXPLANATION
Here we are at Day 2. Reheat the left-over breakfast omelet. Today, you can also reheat last night's dinner for lunch. You already have your easy snacks stashed away at work. Now, remember to have your haddock and kale on hand for dinner time. FYI, the brown rice is optional because you really don't need grains in your meal.

*You will save yourself 108.23 calories by omitting the brown rice from your dinner.

DAY 3

Breakfast
Women: JK Breakfast Omelet (1 serving)

Total Meal Calories: 349.91
Men: JK Breakfast Omelet (1 serving) + Fresh Blueberries (1 cup)
Total Meal Calories: 433.91

Snack 1
Women: JK Avocado Toast (1 serving)
Total Meal Calories: 246.68
Men: JK Avocado Toast (1 serving)
Total Meal Calories: 246.68

Lunch
Women: JK Signature Shake (3/4 serving)
Total Meal Calories: 273.61
Men: JK Signature Shake (1 serving)
Total Meal Calories: 364.81

Snack 2
Women: JK Mixed Nuts (3/4 serving)
Total Meal Calories: 166.05
Men: JK Mixed Nuts (1.5 servings)
Total Meal Calories: 332.10

Dinner
Women: JK Salmon with Asparagus and (optional) Brown Rice (1/2 serving)
Total Meal Calories: 213.90
Men: JK Salmon with Asparagus and (optional) Brown Rice (3/4 serving)
Total Meal Calories: 320.85

Women Total Calories per Day: 1,250.15

Men Total Calories per Day: 1,698.35

EXPLANATION

On Day 3, reheat what's left from your omelet and eat it for breakfast. Blend up a JK Signature Shake for a quick and easy lunch. Have your avocado toast for breakfast, as a snack or even for lunch - whatever fits your schedule best because all of your meals and snacks are interchangeable.

DAY 4

Breakfast
Women: JK Signature Shake (1 serving)
Total Meal Calories: 364.81
Men: JK Signature Shake (1 serving) + Ghee (1 tsp.)
Total Meal Calories: 454.81

Snack 1
Women: JK Carrots with Hummus (2 servings)
Total Meal Calories: 259.44
Men: JK Carrots with Hummus (2 servings)
Total Meal Calories: 259.44

Lunch
Women: JK Salmon with Asparagus and (optional) Brown Rice (1/2 serving)
Total Meal Calories: 213.90
Men: JK Salmon with Asparagus and (optional) Brown Rice (1 serving)
Total Meal Calories: 427.81

Snack 2
Women: JK Green Smoothie (3/4 serving)
Total Meal Calories: 195.78
Men: JK Green Smoothie (1 serving)
Total Meal Calories: 261.05

Dinner
Women: JK Chicken Stir Fry (1 serving)
Total Meal Calories: 216.41
Men: JK Chicken Stir Fry (1.5 servings)
Total Meal Calories: 324.62

Women Total Calories per Day: 1,250.34

Men Total Calories per Day: 1,727.73

EXPLANATION
On Day 4, make two shakes either the night before or first thing in the morning and cover them as quickly as possible so the oxygen doesn't destroy the nutrition. Making these shakes beforehand will cut down on your prep time and cleanup time. Your dinner from the previous night is going to be your lunch, and now all you have to worry about is prepping dinner.

DAY 5

Breakfast
Women: JK Signature Shake (1 serving)
Total Meal Calories: 364.81
Men: JK Signature Shake (1 serving) + ½ avocado (blend it with your shake or eat it on its own)
Total Meal Calories: 525.61

Snack 1
Women: JK Coconut Milk Yogurt with Ground Flaxseed
Total Meal Calories: 204.76
Men: JK Coconut Milk Yogurt with Ground Flaxseed
Total Meal Calories: 204.76

Lunch
Women: JK Chicken Stir Fry (1.5 servings)
Total Meal Calories: 324.62
Men: JK Chicken Stir Fry (2 servings)
Total Meal Calories: 432.82

Snack 2
Women: JK Smashed Avocado (1/2 serving)
Total Meal Calories: 166.68
Men: JK Smashed Avocado (1/2 serving)
Total Meal Calories: 166.68

Dinner
Women: JK Pork with Apple (1 serving)
Total Meal Calories: 224.91
Men: JK Pork with Apple (1.5 servings)
Total Meal Calories: 337.37

Women Total Calories per Day: 1,285.78

Men Total Calories per Day: 1,667.24

EXPLANATION
On Day 5, make your JK Signature Shake first thing in the morning and have your two convenient snacks ready and waiting! What you had for dinner last night is going to be your lunch. You can also use almond milk yogurt in place of the coconut-milk, but make sure it has less than 15 grams of sugar per container.

CONCLUSION
If you are doing this with a significant other, a male is eating the same foods as a female would. The only difference is that the male is increasing the serving size and/or adding food to a meal.

THE TAKE HOME

Any meal - breakfast, lunch, or dinner - can be substituted with the "Create Your Own JK Salad" found at www.ItsFatLossNotWeightLoss.com. If you would like to accelerate weight loss even more, substitute all of your starches, such as brown rice and quinoa, with two additional servings of greens or a small Create Your Own JK Salad. Additionally, if you have any sensitivity to sugar, you can substitute any of the fruit with more vegetables in the smoothies, use extra nuts for the snacks, have another quarter of an avocado instead of half, or skip the rice bread. This will help if you're struggling with your hunger, and you will receive slightly better weight loss results if you are severely insulin sensitive.

The most important part of this whole program is to eat foods that match your preferences AND fall within the guidelines. Keep in mind that the food industries have probably hijacked your taste buds with artificial flavor enhancers and an overload of salt, fat and sugar, so give it time and something you hated before could turn into your new favorite food! The only way you'll want to stick with this program is if you enjoy it. You'll see the best results once you start to have fun by matching it to your preferences. If you eat foods that you hate, your brain will sense that it's missing pleasure. NOT GOOD when you are trying to stick to a program for the long-run. Your brain works to avoid pain and seek out pleasure. If you continue to force down foods that you hate, you will be more likely to overeat the wrong foods and blow the program altogether! All of these meals are not only easy and convenient, but the ingredients can pretty much be purchased almost anywhere. The main goal is to provide you with lifetime results, but the even better part is for you to enjoy it the whole way!

Lifestyle Scale	DESCRIPTION
Serving Size 1 Person Makes 1 Lifetime Result	**Difficulty** – It is **easy** to choose a less **healthy** meal, but sometimes difficult to maintain limits.
Grade Per Person	
Grade	
	Time to Implement – It is only **one meal** on **one day** of the week.
Grade*	
Difficulty 1	**Importance** – You **do not** even **need** to implement this aspect, although it's useful in keeping yourself happy and motivated on your way to achieving long lasting results.
Time to Implement 1 Day	
Importance 3	
*Amount is based off of the average person. Your personal results may be higher or lower depending on your specific needs.	

11

Cheat meals

You may or may not have heard of these things called "cheat meals." Although many dieters allow their cheat **meal** to slowly transition into a cheat **day**, they can be a useful crutch.

WHAT IS A CHEAT MEAL?

If you have been STRICTLY following along with the program for three weeks and making solid changes to your diet, then you **can** have **one** "cheat meal" per week. This meal is meant for you to enjoy a less healthy or unhealthy food or drink that you have been avoiding. First of all, enjoy it, and secondly, don't feel guilty when you see the empty plate. Have that steak and fries with a small slice of pie, but just make sure to enjoy every bite since this is meant to be a morale booster. Of course, if you have a food allergy such as gluten or dairy, you should still stay away from those foods. Just be sure to keep the cheat MEAL to only **one** meal on **one** day and only **once** per week!

WHY CHEAT MEALS?

So, why can this be beneficial? Well, a boost in food intake will put a brief halt to your body being calorie deficient for such a long period of time. The meal gives you **an enjoyable break** from the deficit in calories and that feeling of being deprived from the food you love. Long term deprivation can sneak up on you, and **this cheat meal will lower your chances of binge eating** in the long run because of the food pleasure you are receiving. Being able to look forward to this meal will help you to stick to the diet and keep you pushing toward your ultimate goal.

It's helpful to think about your week as a whole. For instance, think of your friend's birthday party coming up next week, and use that as the opportunity to plan your cheat meal. That way you can go to the birthday party without worry or guilt or acting rude by refusing dessert when your friend is shoving the tray of food in front of your face saying, "Take one!" You should also lower your carbohydrate intake slightly on your cheat meal day. This way you can have that cheat meal but still be semi-conservative on your total carbohydrate intake throughout the day.

Like I said before, I want you to actually enjoy the program while you are on your way to your dream physique. This program isn't meant for you to suffer - it's built so that you CAN and WILL sustain a healthy lifestyle. Taking all the information provided to you in this book and utilizing it will lead you to your dream goals. I hope that you take the education and run with it. Literally!

*The Rant: Many people think they are going to have to stop eating their favorite food forever when they start a fat loss program, but the truth is that you can still have your favorite unhealthy foods as long as you have control over your cheat meals.

Lifestyle Scale	DESCRIPTION
Serving Size 1 Person Makes 1 Lifetime Result	**Difficulty** – For people who do not already do so, starting will be difficult **at first** but **easier** as it goes on.
Grade Per Person	
Grade	
	Grade*	
Difficulty 5	**Time to Implement** – It takes 21 days to **create** or **replace** a habit.
Time to Implement 21 Days	**Importance** – Breakfast will set you up for your **entire day** with **crucial** energy.
Importance 7	
*Amount is based off of the average person. Your personal results may be higher or lower depending on your specific needs.	

12

Eat breakfast!

Eating breakfast increases your metabolism, improves your memory, your mood and your concentration. Eating a solid breakfast will lay the foundation for both your body and mind to wake up and get going, which means fewer groggy mornings that last into groggy afternoons. You really should be trying to eat about 30 minutes after waking up in order to get your metabolism going. If you treat your body right by providing it with what it needs immediately in the morning, it will return the favor by giving you tons of energy!

People sometimes feel like they can't eat anything in the morning or feel sick if they do. This feeling of sickness is most common for people who ate really late the night before, which happens to be horrible for your waistline, by the way. You really shouldn't be eating anything three hours prior to bedtime.

You should eat like a king in the morning, a prince at noon and a pauper at night because your body can process, digest and assimilate nutrients better during the day than at night. Plus, you'll be using these calories during your normal daily activity. Thus, eating breakfast will help you to not overeat at night.

BREAKFAST SETS UP YOUR DAY

Eating a well-balanced breakfast will set the stage for the remainder of your day. Adding protein to your breakfast will further boost your satisfaction through an increased sense of fullness, which of course will reduce your appetite.[1] There are also studies like the "Second Meal Hypothesis," which shows that by eating some complex carbohydrates, instead of ingesting sugar-filled food at breakfast, will improve your glucose tolerance at the next meal.[2] The second meal refers to lunch, so the study showed that people can be insulin sensitive at lunchtime from either skipping breakfast or not eating the correct foods at breakfast. Long-term effects could be insulin resistance and type II diabetes, which, aside from being horrible diseases, also reduce your fat loss efficiency.

HUNGER CHASING

"Hunger chasing" is when you create a nutrient deficiency in your body by skipping breakfast. Your willpower is the highest in the morning and it slowly tapers down as the day progresses. At lunch, your willpower is still at a high level, so you either eat a small meal or don't eat at all, causing even more nutrient deficiencies. By the time the late afternoon hits you're STARVING. This will either cause you to search for something quick to eat, or wait until dinner time. Once you hit dinner, you are so nutrient deficient that you are going to eat everything in sight and your body will never be satisfied. This will also cause you to eat late at night without ever feeling truly full.

*The Rant: Not only does eating breakfast activate your metabolism, but it also helps you to avoid chasing your hunger later in the day.

Lifestyle Scale	DESCRIPTION
Serving Size 1 Person Makes 1 Lifetime Result	**Difficulty –** It is difficult to **judge** liquid calories.
Grade Per Person	
Grade	**Time to Implement –** It takes 21 days to **create** or **replace** a habit.
Grade*	
Difficulty 5	**Importance – Choosing** the right liquids will **skyrocket** your metabolism.
Time to Implement 21 Days	
Importance 8	
*Amount is based off of the average person. Your personal results may be higher or lower depending on your specific needs.	

13

Liquid calories

Water is critical when it comes to losing strictly fat. Water is about 60% of an adult person's body weight. It's the body's main transporter where it acts as a solvent, participates in chemical reactions, provides lubrication and regulates your body's temperature.[1] Use "reverse osmosis" water filters or glass bottled water certified as pure. Additionally, it's probably a no-brainer, but avoid drinking water that is cloudy in any way.

Now, most people think that bottled "spring" water is the healthy way to go, but beware because the Food and Drug Administration (FDA) regulates bottled water companies, while the Environmental Protection Agency (EPA) regulates your tap water. The big deal here is that the FDA has fewer regulations for monitoring water. For example, the FDA doesn't require bottled water companies to test for certain harmful parasites that can affect people with weakened immune systems and the elderly. Horrible, right?

There was also a four-year study done by the National Resources Defense Council where they found that, "Bottled water regulations are inadequate to assure consumers of either purity or safety."[2] So you have to remember that the EPA has regulations that test for harmful parasites to make sure that your water is coming clean to your house, but your store bought bottled "spring" water doesn't even guarantee that it's coming from a pure spring. Gross!

I always recommend glass containers because plastic ones might contain these things called phthalates, which can leach into the water and make it toxic. Phthalates are the chemicals that give plastic its flexibility, but have also been shown to damage the endocrine system, lower testosterone hormones, estrogen hormones and lead to weight gain in the long-run when ingested.[3] So choose glass over plastic when you can. And if you can't, then choose hard plastic over soft plastic.

DEHYDRATION

Dehydration is a major health issue since water is our bodies' single most important fluid that it needs in order to properly function.

Water:

- Protects vital organs
- Assists in homeostasis, which keeps your body in synchronization
- Is a driving force in nutrient absorption
- Keeps your blood volume ideal for exercise performance
- Helps to eliminate toxins

An average adult woman should consume around 2.2L or **9 cups** of water daily.

An average adult man should consume around 3L or **13 cups** of water daily.

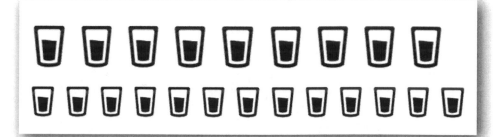

HOW CAN YOU MAKE DRINKING WATER NOT SO "BORING"?

- Add cucumber, lemon, lime, orange slices, crushed berries or boiled ginger to it
- Mix in mint, lemon grass and parsley
- Drink unsweetened tea like black, green, white and rooibos
- Drink sparkling water

When I say sparkling water, I mean top-quality brands like Perrier and San Pellegrino, who sell their water in glass bottles. I would definitely recommend that you stay away from the flavored versions at the convenience store because most of them use artificial flavorings. Furthermore, you should know that there is a HUGE difference between tonic water and club soda. Tonic water has around 23 grams of added sugar and 90 calories in one serving. Club soda, on the other hand, has no sugar and zero calories. Just knowing this can make an ENORMOUS difference in making strides toward your success.

SPORTS DRINKS

The media has blown up sports drinks to make people think they're something that the average individual can consume all day as a healthy alternative to water. Well, hate to break it to you, but they aren't! The only people who really benefit from them are SERIOUS athletes because of the loads of sugar and other ingredients.

Electrolytes, which are the biggest selling points for sports drinks, are made up of a couple of different minerals, but the main one that you need is sodium. Sodium is critical to preventing hypernatremia, which is a condition that leads to water build-up in the brain due to a lack of salt. This condition is most prevalent in athletes who are training **extremely vigorously** for marathons and other high-intensity exercises that cause them to **sweat excessively**, which causes them to lose too much salt.[4]

If you take part in an intense activity lasting for 60-90 minutes, then I would definitely recommend that you replenish your electrolytes[5]. For any activity lasting 90-120 minutes, I recommend that you replenish both your electrolytes as well as your carbohydrates.[5] The reason that these sports drinks contain so much sugar is to replenish athletes with carbs after they have burned through all the glucose in their blood stream. The immediate sugar rush helps replenish stored carbohydrates in the liver and muscles, which gives them energy and aids in recovery. You should note that most of these sports drinks also contain artificial sweeteners, which can cause or contribute to negative health effects as well.

Instead of reaching for a sports drink, make your own by using a fresh lemon, lime, sugar and sea salt. You can find a few recipes online. Coconut water is natural, has a lower calorie count and contains necessary electrolytes and simple sugars to aid in recovering from intense sports performance.

JUICING

Juicing has recently been spreading rapidly through the health industry. While fruit is healthy, of course, drinking only fruit juice instead of eating the whole fruit can be a liquid calorie trap that can also unwittingly rob you of necessary fiber and other nutrients.

Very rarely do the juices that you find in supermarkets contain the fruit that they claim. Mostly, the juice is comprised of water, artificial flavor and a MASSIVE amount of sugar.

It isn't even good enough to make your juices at home. You cut out all the unhealthy additives that processed juices contain, but you're stripping the fiber straight from the whole foods and leaving the drink with sugar and few vitamins. For example, orange juice has the same amount of sugar as a bottle of soda. Downing a glass of fruit juice in a short period of time will create a massive spike in your blood sugar, resulting in a large insulin release. Having these intense sugar spikes is associated with many diseases such as obesity, type II diabetes and cardiovascular disease.

The fiber, vitamins and minerals contained in these foods are meant to be eaten whole and your body WILL know the difference. So do yourself a favor and eat the whole food instead of trying to drink it out of convenience.

COFFEE

Small amounts of coffee can be a healthy choice, but adding heavy cream and sugar will turn this beverage into a nutritional nightmare.

Organic coffee taken black provides you with anti-oxidants that help clean up your body. Additionally, the caffeine will not only wake you up, but it can also enhance your cognition, increase your athletic performance and aid in fighting fat.[4] Caffeine increases your body's metabolic rate, which in turn helps you burn more calories throughout the day.

What you need to know is that not all coffee is created equal! Adding two sugars and a cream is just the start of many ways we can go wrong ordering from our favorite barista. For example, Dunkin Donuts' large

Frozen Caramel Coffee Coolatta with cream breaks the scale, weighing in at **1,050 calories**! That's right, 1,050 calories for just one drink! By contrast, a cup of regular black coffee comes in at just **2 calories**!

The large Frozen Caramel Coffee Coolatta with cream contains 52 grams of fat, which is almost double the amount of fat in a Big Mac from McDonald's! How much sugar you ask? It contains 130 grams of sugar, which is the same as eating a **full pint** of Ben & Jerry's Phish Food Ice Cream! If you drink one of these every day, you could be gaining 2 pounds of fat per week.

Now can you see where making the switch to black coffee with some almond milk or stevia is going to save tons of liquid calories? This type of coffee only costs you under 50 calories and literally saves you 1,000 calories per day, but remember that caffeine is still a drug. Your body has to metabolize it in order to reap the benefits, and when it's taken in excessive amounts it can be more harmful than beneficial.

SODA & DIET SODA

We all know that soda is bad for us, but how bad is it honestly? Well, it's REALLY, REALLY BAD! Soda has pretty much all of the same properties as putting sugar in carbonated water. A lot of sugar ingested in a short period of time leads to that terrible condition we know as insulin resistance. Sodas have no nutritional value, and the Center for Science refers to them as "liquid candy." If you have been reading through this book, you should know by now that a lot of sugar with little or no fiber will lead to TONS of problems down the road. Soda has absolutely no health benefits at all, so stay away from it! This goes double for giving it to your children!

A 16 oz. bottle of soda can have just as much caffeine as a cup of coffee. Couple that with the amount of added sugar in the soda and this is the worst nutritional option to offer any child. Children's bodies are not designed to handle caffeine at such a young age. Not only will they be off the walls then immediately down for the count, but the intense amount of sugar can lead to health problems in the future.

You might be wondering about diet soda since some of these don't even have any calories. In the past 20 years, it has been shown that drinking diet colas is just as bad as drinking regular cola when it comes to weight gain. There has yet to be a study that shows long-term weight loss from consuming these diet drinks. And the artificial sweeteners in these beverages cause negative side effects plain and simple.

There are three reasons why you should stop drinking artificial sweeteners.[7,8]

1. They mimic insulin; therefore they cause your metabolism to slow down by not allowing your body to burn fat for energy.
2. They increase your LDL or bad cholesterol due to insulin resistance.
3. They increase your hunger.

People have GAINED weight while drinking these.

Dr. Mark Hyman, a practicing functional medicine doctor, found that those who consume diet drinks regularly have a 200 percent increased risk of weight gain, a 36 percent increased risk of pre-diabetes or metabolic syndrome, and a 67 percent increased risk of diabetes[5].

Some of these drinks are extremely addictive, so when you're trying to eliminate diet or regular colas from your life, remember you have to replace both the caffeine and carbonation. Try replacing the caffeine with black coffee, green tea or black tea. To replace the bubbly, try drinking seltzer water instead – you can buy them from your local wholesaler by the case. You can also get creative by putting any of the cold caffeine recommendations in with the bubbly water. It's truly fantastic!

ALCOHOL

I recommend that you stay away from alcohol as much as possible because of the amount of empty calories in it.

If you've heard that drinking red wine makes you healthier, you should know that you'd have to drink 40 liters of red wine each day in order to reap the benefits of resveratrol and anti-oxidants![9] Wine also has more calories than most alcoholic drinks, so there are some better options out there. Don't get me wrong, wine is still better than drinking a margarita, but just watch how much you are taking in.

*Resveratrol: a compound produced by several plants, which is thought to have antioxidant properties, protecting the body against an increased risk of heart disease and cancer.

Stick to the clear alcohols such as tequila, white rum, vodka or gin. If you need a mixer for any of your drinks, choose seltzer water and a slice of fruit for a garnish over sodas or fruit juices. Remember to stay away from tonic water though! If you want to be bold, using just normal water as a mixer would be better yet. Not only does water have zero calories, but it will also counteract alcohol's dehydration effect.

*There are a few **gluten-free** alcoholic beverages on the market which are highly recommended, but make sure to do your research!

*The Rant: Most liquids are silent calorie traps – choosing water will always be your best bet, but making better choices with other liquids will help you receive increased fat loss.

Lifestyle Scale	DESCRIPTION
Serving Size 1 Person Makes 1 Lifetime Result	**Difficulty –** Properly **dosing** caffeine without becoming **addicted** is the key.
Grade Per Person	
Grade	
Grade*	**Time to Implement –** It takes 21 days to **create** or **replace** a habit.
Difficulty 5	
Time to Implement 21 Days	**Importance –** You don't need caffeine, but **supplementing** it can help you **burn fat**.
Importance 3	
*Amount is based off of the average person. Your personal results may be higher or lower depending on your specific needs.	

14

What does caffeine do?

Caffeine can be used as a drug, for food or – as many athletes ingest it - as a dietary supplement. Believe it or not, it's the most widely consumed "behaviorally active" substance in the world, which just means it's a chemical that causes a reaction in your body.

When you ingest caffeine, your intestinal tract absorbs it rapidly to give you a very quick response, which is commonly called a "caffeine high," which extends your endurance in strenuous aerobic exercise like running and also in shorter duration maximal effort like weight training.

CAFFEINE'S MECHANISM FOR ACTION

Ingesting caffeine within an hour of working out will help your body burn fat because it spares your stored energy in your liver and muscles, which are critical during any aerobic or anaerobic training session. Instead, caffeine causes your body to use your fat as a primary exercise fuel[1]. Sparing these liver and muscle reserves especially benefits prolonged high-intensity exercise by increasing your endurance.[1,2]

Caffeine fights fat in two ways:[1,2]

1. It works by drawing energy **directly** from your adipose tissues (fat) and peripheral vascular tissues.
2. It indirectly stimulates an epinephrine release by the adrenal medulla, meaning simply that your body will release adrenaline into the bloodstream.

CAFFEINE WARNINGS

Although caffeine consumption clearly has some fat loss benefits, it doesn't mean that you should drink five cups of coffee or take three scoops of pre-workout before exercising. And it certainly doesn't mean that you should chug soda since the amount of sugar in it would counteract the positive effects of the caffeine and cause health problems on top of that.

Black coffee works the best, but if you need to add something, put in a splash of almond milk and some stevia for a zero-calorie natural sweetener. Adding cream or sugar would, as with soda, simply counteract the health benefits.

Like anything else in life, with the positives, unfortunately always come the negatives. The effects from caffeine become less apparent if you consume a high-carbohydrate diet or if you use caffeine habitually. Your body will eventually get used to the caffeine and the effects will taper off slowly.

Here are some doom and gloom effects of caffeine.

Caffeine can cause.[1,2]

- Restlessness
- Headaches
- Insomnia
- Nervous irritability
- Muscle twitching
- Tremulousness
- Psychomotor agitation
- Elevated heart rate
- Elevated blood pressure
- Premature left ventricular contractions

Don't freak out and throw out all of your coffee. Many of these effects are caused by an extreme dose of caffeine, but everyone is different. If you are experiencing some of these side effects, you may want to consult with your doctor and see what is going on. Your body might not be able to handle the amount of caffeine that you're ingesting.

Caffeine also acts as a diuretic. This means that it will cause you to urinate more often. This could cause unnecessary pre-exercise loss of fluid that negatively affects your thermal balance and exercise performance, especially in a hot environment. Basically, you'll dehydrate faster so you'll have to remember to stock up on the water and stay hydrated.

THE VERDICT ON CAFFEINE

So what's the final verdict? Caffeine is addictive and it can tax your adrenal glands when used excessively, which can lead to fatigue. This is especially true when you are already taxing your adrenal glands in other ways such as being stressed, chronically overtraining or not getting enough quality sleep. Additionally, caffeine is NOT recommended for children or adolescents. That being said, if you are consuming coffee daily and would like to use caffeine as a supplement for any type of training or exercise, drink some 45 minutes prior to exercising. This can aid you in body fat loss and enhance your endurance while training, but it's vital that you remain extremely cautious while consuming it. The maximum dose of caffeine before a workout is 250mg, which is around 2 cups of brewed coffee. Like I said before, don't go and ingest as much caffeine as you can, but a cup or two of black coffee should help you in reaching some of your fitness goals.

*The Rant: There are both positives and negatives when it comes to caffeine – doing what works for you remains vital in your program

Lifestyle Scale	DESCRIPTION
Serving Size 1 Person Makes 1 Lifetime Result	**Difficulty** – Just **showng up** is the **hardest** part of exercising.
Grade Per Person	
Grade	**Time to Implement** – It takes 21 days to **create** or **replace** a habit.
Grade*	
Difficulty 5	**Importance** – Exercise **boosts** fat loss and is **crucial** in maintaining permanent results.
Time to Implement 21 Days	
Importance 9	
*Amount is based off of the average person. Your personal results may be higher or lower depending on your specific needs.	

15

Exercise

WARNING: You must consult with your doctor prior to performing any type of exercise program. This warning is usually meant for those individuals with extreme heart conditions because the risk of a cardiac-related complication is extremely small for the rest of the population.

Regular exercise will play a CRITICAL role in reducing the amount of fat on your body as well as building LEAN muscle on your frame. More muscle = higher metabolism = less body fat.

JUST SHOW UP

Okay, let's dive in! I like to take a quote from Woody Allen, where he stated, "80% of success is just showing up," and it couldn't be more accurate here. **Any** physical activity performed is worth 1,000x's not doing any at all. Studies have shown that <u>inactivity is just as damaging to a person's health as smoking a pack of cigarettes every day.</u>[1]

Being an ACE Certified Personal Trainer and Health Coach, I am an expert when it comes to anything that involves exercise. It's shown that regular physical activity reduces the risk of tons of damaging health outcomes. Furthermore, you will receive additional benefits as the amount of physical activity increases through higher intensity, more frequency, and longer durations. To a point, of course. Most of these benefits occur with at least 210 minutes (three and a half hours) of moderate-intensity activity each week. That's only 30 minutes per day, so there's really no excuse!

Our bodies were not meant to sit at a desk all day, sit on a couch all evening and then lie down in a bed all night. Our bodies were meant to MOVE!

WHAT KIND OF EXERCISE?

Both aerobic and anaerobic exercise is beneficial to the body. Aerobic physical activity means endurance-type exercises such as long-distance running, biking and rowing. Anaerobic physical activity means your muscle strengthening-type exercises such as weight lifting, sprinting and body-weight exercises.

What's truly amazing is that the health benefits of physical activity happen for everyone, whether you have a disease or a disability, whether you're old or young, and whether you're already living a healthy lifestyle or just beginning to. Just acknowledge that injuries may result from exercising, but this should not dissuade you from exercising because the benefits are so tremendous!

One such amazing benefit is that physical activity also helps you to become more mentally sharp!

The Journal, *NeuroMolecular Medicine*, shows research that clearly proves exercise enhances the cognition of your mind. Furthermore, physical activity is actually more effective in this regard than nutritional supplements, brain training, medications and pharmaceuticals.[2]

EXERCISE CREATES HEALTH

So how does exercise create health? First, it lowers the amount of free radicals in your body, which are responsible for making oxidative stress.[3,4] Oxidative stress is sort of like the rust on a car, but in every cell of your body.

*Free radicals- an uncharged molecule shown to cause damage to the body on the cellular level

Don't get me wrong, free radicals are a normal part of your body's chemistry, but **excessive** free radicals cause cellular damage. This damage can be easily avoided by regularly exercising and practicing the other wellness tips throughout this book.

This regular physical activity is going to enhance your body's performance from the inside of your cells! In every cell, there are mitochondria, which act as "power plants" by converting the food you ingest into a form of useable energy called adenosine triphosphate (ATP). ATP is what allows us to maintain all of our bodily functions, and if the mitochondria are not taken care of, they can malfunction, which causes SERIOUS damage.[4]

INACTIVITY IS THE ENEMY

So what causes this damage? INACTIVITY! You wouldn't think that doing nothing all day could hurt you, but it does. When thinking of your mitochondria think "use it or lose it." Inactivity will cause damage to the mitochondria, eventually leading them to die off. This damage can cause a loss of cellular function, a massive decrease in metabolism, a loss of physical energy and a halt on cellular healing, which leads to the accumulation of toxins within the body. Some of these toxins, like free radicals, will run wild and cause cellular death and disease.

How do you stop this? Easy, you GET MOVING! Exercise is the number one way to not only create new mitochondria, but also to keep your existing mitochondria healthy, which in turn leads to anti-aging effects and an increased metabolism. Even though exercise is the number one way to do all of this, there are SPECIFIC ways to exercise that will lead to these great health benefits.

LIVE AN ACTIVE LIFESTYLE

Your first step is going to be just showing up. Making it to the point that you are actually doing the physical activity is the first part of gaining all of these benefits. Step two is going to be giving it your ALL. Walking is a great start, but actual intensity will provide you with a better return on your investment of time and energy. With time and consistence, pushing yourself will give you the maximum benefits. However, MAKE SURE TO ONLY PUSH TO YOUR OWN ABILITY. Just because you saw someone in the gym doing something doesn't mean that you're prepared to try it. Some people have been exercising for years, so take it slow at first if you're inexperienced or out of practice. Everyone has to start somewhere. Progressing to your body's ability to exercise harder and longer **when you're ready to do so** is when you'll see massive results.

I really like to push anaerobic exercise, which is your higher-intensity physical activity. Warm up a little and try some interval training sprints once or twice a week. This is a series of shorter bouts of high-intensity cardiovascular exercise followed by low-intensity cardiovascular exercise. You can try doing 30 seconds of sprinting your hardest followed by 2 minutes of walking. This is going to get your heart rate to skyrocket and then drop, which is a great way to torch body fat. If you're not the running type, try out a different cardiovascular machine until you find your favorite.

*Even though we are talking about cardiovascular exercise, performing intervals classifies it as anaerobic exercise.

Strength training is another form of anaerobic exercise that is HIGHLY recommended. Performing your compound exercises such as squats, deadlifts and lunges will give you the best results because you are using more muscles at one time, stimulating more of your central nervous system and burning more calories in a lesser amount of time. If you were to "superset" your exercises, which means doing one exercise followed by another exercise that works a different muscle group with no rest in between, you will see **massive** results. Both interval and weight training done together will make your body adapt to the extra stress by increasing the amount of mitochondria in it!

WOMEN NEED WEIGHTS!

Most women get nervous when I tell them to start lifting weights because they "don't want to look like a man." I am here to tell you that YOU WON'T! Women do not have the natural hormones that men do in order to become muscle bound. Weight training will help you to tone up and reduce body fat.

Weight training has been shown to:[5]

- Increase bone density
- Improve muscular strength
- Improve muscle size and shape
- Improve immune system function
- Improve flexibility

PUSH YOURSELF

The harder you push yourself, the faster your metabolism will get. Just like cardio exercise, your heart rate is going to be elevated during weight training. This elevated heart rate will cause Excess Post-Exercise Oxygen Consumption (EPOC), which increases your metabolism and **promotes fat burning for hours after you train**.[6,7]

What you need to know is that the harder you push yourself with anaerobic exercise, the more recovery you are going to need. When you are weight training, this is going to depend on your workout duration, health and muscle soreness, so you should be looking out for signs of over-training, including increased lethargy, restlessness, a decrease in strength or endurance, elevated blood pressure, injury, illness, a lack of motivation and increased soreness. When starting out, performing weight training only a few days a week is a great way to begin your physical activity program.

BE A CARDIO KING/QUEEN

With all of these benefits just from weight training, it's easy to forget about cardio, but cardiovascular training is also going to remain crucial for seeing the best results.

Cardiovascular training has been shown to:[5]

- Improve endurance
- Reduce stress hormones
- Improve heart and lung efficiency
- Improve general health and fitness

The good news is that when it comes to cardio, the more the better! This type of exercise doesn't break down your muscle as much as weight training. The only problem is that it will not build actual muscle or directly tone your muscles. Rather, this is going to be the supplement to your anaerobic-training program.

PERIODIZATION TRAINING

A very heavily marketed term within the fitness industry is the training technique of "muscle confusion." This is a form of training designed to avoid a stall in results by allowing muscle groups to continuously improve during phases of unfamiliar movements. Although muscle confusion is true in certain aspects of training, when it comes to burning fat effectively, there's another term that I like to use instead, which breaks the technique down into more detail.

Instead of using the term "muscle confusion," I like to refer to it as the scientific term, **periodization**. Although both words have similar meanings, their definitions are slightly different. Periodization refers to a **planned** progression of resistance training in which you are intentionally varying the exercise plan, especially in respect to volume and intensity – this has been shown to increase strength and peak performance as compared to standardized resistance training.

*Training volume: How many exercises you are performing in a single session.

You should be changing the types of resistance, amount of reps and amount of sets you are performing if your workouts become stale. However, this doesn't mean that you should be entering the gym without a plan for each and every workout session. Exercise is just as much of a science as nutrition, and without a well-developed exercise plan, it's like you are driving a car without a steering wheel.

When you are performing periodization resistance training, it should be broken up into certain time segments referred to as macrocycles, mesocycles and microcycles. Macrocycles refer to the overall time frame of the training period usually covering anywhere from 6 to 12 months - this is going to be where you set your long-term goal for the overall program. Mesocycles refer to the slightly smaller goals of the macrocycle, typically made in three-month blocks. However, since three months represent a long period of time, mesocycles are broken down even more into the smallest time frame called microcycles. These refer to two to four week goals of the exercise program. I recommend that you schedule these time periods, along with their corresponding goals, on a calendar so that you can see where you stand as progress is made.

FIND YOUR LEVEL

As with anything else in life, everyone has to start somewhere. This means that not everyone is going to be at the same level when it comes to fitness. You could be a beginner, a daily gym-goer or a seasoned veteran. Either way, performing to your ability within your activity level is going to provide you with immense results.

If you are in the beginning stage of working out, I highly recommend that you invest in a personal trainer at your local gym or fitness center. Not only are they going to assess where you stand physically, but they are going to be able to guide you toward your goals step by step. Some people in this stage might have to work on solving stability issues that include posture, flexibility and basic movement of the body before they even think of picking up a weight. Others may be at a level where they feel comfortable hitting the weights right away. Either way, seeking out a personal trainer who you feel comfortable with, has the proper credentials and pushes you to your own abilities will provide you with the extra tools you need in order to accelerate your fat loss.

*Make sure you work with NCCA accredited personal trainers - this is the gold standard for personal training.

If you are a daily gym-goer, but lack experience with regular weight training, I also recommend that you invest in a few sessions with a personal trainer. If you feel that you know the basics, start off easy and progress slowly. Use the periodization training technique that I explained, setting microcycle, mesocycle and macrocycle goals that you want to reach.

For the seasoned veteran, hitting the gym is going to be your favorite part, but remember that your nutrition, mindset and lifestyle choices are going to be equally important. As with the daily gym-goers, I highly recommend that you set goals for yourself using the periodization training technique. This is going to give you a proper plan to follow for years!

APPROPRIATE RATES OF PROGRESSION

Although physical activity remains a very important part of permanent fat loss, make sure that you are not performing at a level that your body cannot handle. I have seen clients who were doing great until they hurt themselves at the gym by attempting to do more weight than their body could handle. Making sure that you progress slowly in the gym is crucial to preventing injury.

Concentrate on nailing down proper form before you even think about increasing the weight. Keeping your movements controlled will not only prevent you from getting injured, but it is also going to provide you with the most benefits of weight training. Try to feel your muscle working while you are performing your exercises. Essentially you should be doing your reps slow and steady instead of trying to blow through them. This will increase stress on the muscle, which is extremely important because your muscle can handle the extra stimulation (that's how they grow). However, if you do not use proper form, your tendons that connect muscle to bone will not uphold unless the movement is controlled – this tends to lead to injury.

Once you are able to **easily** perform the scheduled amount of reps of a single movement at a certain weight for the scheduled amount of sets, you can increase your weight load by 5% depending on the movement. This may not sound like a lot of weight, but your body will feel it once you bump that weight up just a little. The repetitions will become more difficult and you will need to exert more energy in order to complete those reps for multiple sets.

*Resistance increases could be more than 5% if the exerciser is experiencing a fast rate of progression.

As for cardiovascular training, progression is going to be made through the duration and intensity of the physical activity being performed. Duration is the amount of time the cardiovascular exercise is being performed, and intensity is the amount of energy you are using with the same duration of a cardiovascular exercise.

As a beginner, you are going to want to make progressions through increasing the duration of the cardiovascular exercise. These progressions should be made slightly by adding on 30-60 seconds once you are able to complete a cardiovascular exercise for two weeks. I do not recommend that you increase intensity until you are comfortable with performing the exercise - if so, make sure that you only increase the intensity **slightly**.

As a daily gym-goer, you can progress with your cardiovascular exercise by increasing both the duration and intensity of the physical activity. As with the beginners, you should feel completely comfortable with the movement before you increase the intensity of the movement.

As a seasoned veteran, you can also progress by increasing both the duration and intensity of the physical activity. At this level, I highly recommend that you increase the intensity of your movement. This is going to give you the best results when it comes to accelerated fat loss. As with any other type of movement, make sure that you are comfortable with performing it prior to increasing either the duration or intensity.

BUILD LEAN MUSCLE

Since we are looking to burn fat, we should be aiming for muscle hypertrophy. This is the process of muscle-fiber enlargement (gaining more muscle) that results from progressive weight training. The amount of sets, reps, training volume and frequency are critical, but the most important piece is intensity! Intensity isn't about adding more sets or having a longer work out - it's about how much force, power and effort you are putting into working the muscle tissues. Concentrating on stimulating the muscle tissue to the best of your given ability is the goal here. To achieve maximum muscle hypertrophy, this will depend on intensity plus **adequate recovery time**! You should allow a muscle group to recover for 48-72 hours after intensely training it.

*The best way to increase intensity is by remaining mentally focused on the task at hand.

Depending on your exercise level, you are going to want to aim for 3-4 sets of 8-12 reps for each exercise you are performing. However, you should always start at a higher rep range and lighter weight until you get a feel for the muscles you are working. If you are a beginner, I recommend that you use lighter weight, concentrate on form and aim for the higher end of this range, especially if you are taking your muscles to failure. For the more seasoned weight trainers, you can push a little harder and also take your muscles to failure. However, if you choose to push your muscles to the level of failure, it should occur within the rep range of 8-12. This is going to provide you with the best opportunity for muscle hypertrophy, which will in turn lead to a loss of body fat.

FIND THE TIME!

We all have the same 24 hours in each day and, like I said before, you only need to find a minimum of 30 minutes a day to work out. But even when your time is limited, **something** is always better than **nothing**. You can use high intensity or interval training, which increases the number of mitochondria and burns more fat over time from EPOC.

FATS BURN IN THE FLAME OF CARBS

Some people love to do their **high-intensity** training in the early mornings before the day sucks them in (which I recommend). If you choose to do so, you must know that you need to ingest a small amount of carbohydrates from a whole food source at least 60 minutes prior to working out in order for your body to burn fat as energy.

If the body is lacking carbohydrates when performing **intense** physical activity, critical amino acids are stripped out of muscle tissue to be utilized as energy.[6,7] This stripping of the muscle tissue reduces the body's metabolic rate drastically. However, this is only a problem if you are training at a **high intensity** on an empty stomach right after you wake up each day. On the other hand, low-intensity cardio will not use the same energy system, so you can do your low-intensity cardio on an empty stomach.

*Remember, high intensity training will accelerate fat burning!

When looking for something to eat prior to training, make sure it's something that is small and easily digestible. I highly recommend a plant-based smoothie like a quarter of my JK Signature Shake. Not only will it provide you with the necessary amount of carbohydrates for your workout, but it will also give you a substantial amount of nutrients that will set you up for the remainder of your day! Other small recommendations are a tablespoon of almond butter or coconut butter, a piece of fruit or a quarter of an avocado. Like I said before, make sure that you wait an hour for it to digest. If you're rushed for time, cut the portion in half so that you only have to wait 30 minutes. I highly recommend that you play around with different portions and servings in order to see what works best for you.

*Go to www.ItsFatLossNotWeightLoss.com for the most recent Five-Day Breakdown & Recipes

*If you're a coffee drinker, have it 30-45 minutes prior to your workout to gain the extra energy, but make sure to stay hydrated!

WHEN TO DO WHAT

When developing your workout program, should regular resistance training take place before or after cardiovascular training?

When you're ready to exercise, warm up for five to ten minutes with some light cardio, which will get your body out of the parasympathetic drive (your rest and digest mode) and into the sympathetic drive (your fight or flight mode). The ONLY time you are going to want to be in fight or flight mode is during physical activity because this is when your body is going to switch itself into being the most effective at using glycogen for energy, which is the best energy source for building lean muscle.[8,9]

So after you warm up and get into the sympathetic drive, you should hit the weights HARD so your body uses up its glycogen storage. Once your glycogen storage is depleted and your body is ready to start using fat as energy, you'll finish up your workout with some high-intensity cardiovascular exercise, which is the most proficient at torching fat.[5,6]

*The body always uses a mixture of both fat and carbohydrates for energy. While training, the body is going to rely mostly on carbohydrates for energy.

In summary, to burn the most fat:

- Warm up with light cardio
- Hit the weights HARD
- Finish with more intense cardio
- Burn fat
- Feel good

You get it, right?

DO I REALLY HAVE TO STRETCH?

Stretching prevents injury, improves your flexibility, reduces muscle soreness and helps promote muscle building![5] Your muscles are surrounded by fascia, which is a strong connective tissue that provides structure and protection. When you stretch the fascia, you allow room for your muscles to grow – but make sure to never stretch a cold muscle! Stretching before workouts can actually cause injury and decrease performance because there is a lack of blood flow to your muscles.[8,9] The best time to stretch is directly following your workout focusing mainly on the muscle group you have trained.

MIND-BODY PHYSICAL ACTIVITY

Performed both as individual and group workouts, mind-body exercises are great low-to-moderate intensity physical activities that help to strengthen both the body and mind. As I said before, any type of exercise is good for the mind, but specific types such as yoga, tai chi, Pilates and qigong are a few examples that concentrate on strengthening strictly the mind-body connection.

*There have been thousands of published research articles written about mind-body exercises proving them to be beneficial to the body.

The major difference between traditional forms of exercise like weight training and running compared to mind-body is that traditional exercise is centered on physical goals such as measurements of body fat or lifting a set amount of weight. Mind-body exercises are centered upon your perceived effort, specific breathing techniques and self-awareness. When performed properly, mind-body exercises can halt the progression of diseases such as arthritis, diabetes and cardiovascular disease.

*Tai Chi has been shown to reduce anxiety, symptoms of depression and blood pressure.

Although a very difficult type of exercise to master, remember that different types of mind-body exercises can vary in the amount of calories you burn each session. Don't just rely on this type of exercise in order to see major fat loss results. However, supplementing it with your traditional aerobic and anaerobic exercises can be beneficial to your program.

GET YOUR N.E.A.T. ON

N.E.A.T. (**N**on-**E**xercise **A**ctivity **T**hermogenesis) is going to be your typical daily activity like standing, moving, walking, gardening or dancing. At work, you can sit on a yoga ball, use a standing desk, have a walking meeting or anything else that will get you moving more. I recommend that all of this be performed up to 2.5 hours each day.

* N.E.A.T. is a daily movement, NOT exercise! These types of movements will not increase your metabolism or secrete the hormones that burn fat.

FIND YOUR WORKOUT

There isn't one "right" way to exercise and there's no such thing as a "perfect" workout. The fact of the matter is that our bodies adapt to our environments and our activities, so it'll be important for you to create different workouts that will continue to challenge and stimulate your body.

I told you to do what you are capable of, but another HUGE aspect of this is going to rely on what you actually LIKE. Exercise should be **fun**, not a chore. Have some fun with it by switching it up sometimes. If you hate a certain type of exercise, **do something else**! There is always going to be something out there for you that you will enjoy. So go out, find it and DO IT!

Remember these tips when it comes to exercise:

* If you do something every day, it will become habit!
* Train harder
* Make it fun
* And just show up!

*The Rant: There are so many different ways to exercise your body, so find what you enjoy the most. Challenging your body will come naturally after you find an activity that you enjoy.

Lifestyle Scale	DESCRIPTION
Serving Size 1 Person Makes 1 Lifetime Result	**Difficulty** – It will be difficult to implement **every** aspect of wellness.
Grade Per Person	
Grade	**Time to Implement** – Wellness is an **ongoing** practice to get **better** at.
Grade*	
Difficulty 10	
Time to Implement Never Ending	**Importance** – Implementing as many aspects of wellness as
Importance 10	**possible** will lead to **permanent** results.
*Amount is based off of the average person. Your personal results may be higher or lower depending on your specific needs.	

16

Wellness

Few people really know that the progression of most diseases, including obesity, can actually be halted. Or that many conditions can be reversed through the right diet and lifestyle changes[1, 2]. A healthy lifestyle can reduce the degree of poor health that most people have to endure at the end of their lives, which will improve quality of life, extend independence and reduce time spent in hospitals or otherwise receiving medical treatment. But there are benefits to reap even before you reach your twilight years. Wellness can help you live a high-quality active life until the very end. We should all want to live a happy life, right? Not suffering from degenerative disease or having to go to doctors' offices to undergo horrible treatments.

We all have genetic differences that affect our health, but these genetic expressions are outweighed by our health habits. Habits such as diet and lifestyle choices, whether those choices are good or bad, will determine which genetic expression reacts, including "turning on" chronic illnesses. I like to tell people that genetics loads the gun and your environment pulls the trigger! The good news is that, collectively, excellent wellness will translate to overall health, and health has a direct correlation with weight loss!

*Environment: When I say, "your environment pulls the trigger," I mean the poor-quality foods, biased information and the hustle & bustle society that we are surrounded by.

SORT THROUGH THE CONTRADICTIONS

It can be difficult knowing how best to achieve health and wellness because many companies use aggressive marketing tactics that can make it difficult for the public to separate fact from fiction. It's difficult even for scientists using the best tools available to discover the truth about good health, and in fact there are often contradictory findings!

As an example, let's take the "findings" on eggs and the correlation that they have with health. This week it could be that you should be eating eggs every day, and the following week new findings will tell you that the cholesterol in eggs causes heart disease (which is false), and you should stop eating them. What the media doesn't tell you is what is most important, which is that the quality of eggs that you eat is really what matters. For example, free-range eggs have five times the amount of anti-inflammatory fat compared to conventional eggs[3]. Both are called "eggs," but in reality they affect your body drastically differently.

WHAT IS WELLNESS?

Now, let's get back to this word, "wellness." What does it mean? The easiest way that I can explain wellness to you is by showing you my "Wellness

Wheel" diagram. I call this a Wellness "Wheel" because if there are any imperfections in the perfectly circular shape while it's rolling, there are going to be problems. Also, no one point is further away from the center compared to another, meaning that each point is just as important as the last. So when you think of wellness, think of it being the center of your circle and everything around it is what's protecting it.

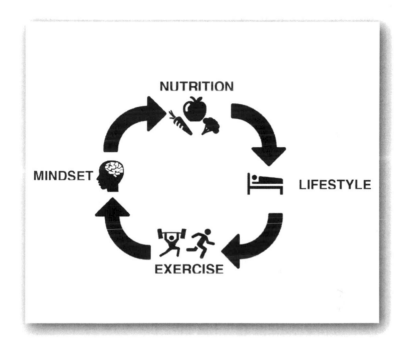

As you can see, there are four MAIN aspects when it comes to wellness: nutrition, lifestyle, exercise and mindset. In general terms, **nutrition** represents quality foods, portion control and meal timing. **Lifestyle** includes sleep hygiene, stress management and social interactions. **Exercise** includes your physical activities, the amount of daily movement and physical hobbies. **Mindset** includes your thought patterns, willpower and meditation.

*Physical hobbies: These are less-intense hobbies like gardening, fishing, light yard work, etc.

Like I said before, when we look at wellness, each aspect of this Wellness Wheel remains equally important. If you are eating properly but stressed every day, your results can actually be negated. If you are exercising six days a week, but eating junk food all day and night, you won't see the results you are expecting. Furthermore, if you are sitting all day and never getting up to move, your body is not going to respond very well.

DO WHAT YOU ARE CAPABLE OF

It's definitely not going to be easy, but as you practice each of these aspects every day, you are going to get better and better at them until you become your own master of true wellness. Even if that means taking small steps toward mastering these skills, you will achieve lasting results in time.

I have no cartilage under my right knee and have had massive shoulder reconstruction. My body is no longer built to run a marathon or to perform Olympic lifts over my head. Therefore, I am not able to do what I used to, but there are several alternatives that I CAN do, and knowing what I AM capable of doing is a driving factor for me. This knowledge leads me to not only do the activities that I'm still capable of, but to always strive to do them better every single day. Whether I'm meditating, exercising, increasing productivity at work or most importantly being a father, my dedication to excellence is immense. And health and wellness is no different because it's something that you must practice for a long time, and you might not ever master it completely. Just remember that showing up every day is the key. As Aristotle said over a thousand years ago, "We are what we repeatedly do. Excellence, then, is not an act, but a habit." So do something to contribute to your health and wellness day after day, and then year after year. You will achieve excellence in what you have set out to do!

*The Rant: When it comes to wellness, there are so many factors to keep in mind in order to attain permanent results – the most important part is to implement as many as you can in your life, which will lead you toward ultimate success!

Lifestyle Scale	DESCRIPTION
Serving Size 1 Person Makes 1 Lifetime Result	**Difficulty** – Attaining any **goal** requires hard work and **dedication**.
Grade Per Person	
Grade	
Grade*	**Time to Implement** – It takes 21 days to **create** or **replace** a habit.
Difficulty 4	
Time to Implement 21 Days	**Importance** – It is important to set up **realistic** goals which will lead you toward **ultimate** goals.
Importance 4	
*Amount is based off of the average person. Your personal results may be higher or lower depending on your specific needs.	

17

Goals

It's crucial to set **realistic** goals where you understand what the obstacles in your way to success **really** are. It can be tempting to focus solely on plowing through your goals from beginning to end, but taking a step back and creating an effective strategy can save you time and energy. Think of it as the difference between going around a mountain rather than going up and over it. You want to work smarter, not harder. Because if you exhaust yourself halfway up or even around that mountain with unrealistic goals and expectations, then you're going to feel disheartened when you fail – and you will have in fact set yourself up for failure.

*If you put all of your effort into following the program instead of hitting your specific goal, not only will the goal come as a side effect, but you will also drastically reduce your stress level.

START SMALL

I recommend aiming for making smaller, more easily attainable goals to achieve. Set a goal to get a third of the way up or around that mountain rather than all the way up and over in one go. Keep in mind that if you don't believe in yourself, you will never make it to any goal that you set, no matter how hard you try. So only undertake goals that you believe that you can achieve.

What you might not know is that 40% of our daily actions aren't decisions, but habits. Habits allow the brain to conserve energy and circumvent overstimulation. Understanding your habits will help you to reach your goals more easily.

When modifying habits, it is best to focus on only **one at a time**. Make the change **real** by believing in yourself and the reason you're making this change. Next, you must determine and identify your routine by journaling any of your triggers that may cause a relapse into your old habits.

STAY REALISTIC

Willpower plays an enormous role in the success or failure of your goal setting, too. Willpower is a skill, and as with any skill, it requires time and hard work to develop it. Willpower is also a finite, though replenishable, resource, which is why it's **critical** to set **realistic** goals. Because **unrealistic goals** will exhaust your willpower in the short term and discourage you from setting out to achieve other goals in the future. Just keep in mind that we're all snowflakes, so you'll likely need to try different techniques until you discover the ones that work SPECIFICALLY for you.

I frequently recommend the sandwich technique, which is just setting a small goal that piggybacks onto something familiar. This is an effective strategy because you can focus on a small goal more easily and without having to make a drastic change to your current habits. For instance, if you eat eggs every morning, simply adding vegetables to create an omelet will create a healthier meal. If you like to eat chicken noodle soup every day, replace the noodles with spaghetti squash or another type of vegetable. If you like to eat pita bread and hummus for a snack, replace the pita bread with celery and carrots to dip into the hummus.

These small changes are a great way to get started in the right direction to achieve any kind of goal, including health-related goals such as fat loss. It's never easy changing a habit completely, but using these small changes will add up to the bigger changes down the road that you'll ultimately need to attain your goals.

*The Rant: Creating small, attainable goals which you can reach will lead you toward accomplishing your much larger goals in the long-run.

Lifestyle Scale	DESCRIPTION
Serving Size 1 Person Makes 1 Lifetime Result	**Difficulty** – It may be difficult to
Grade Per Person	**start** meditating, but will get **easier**
Grade	as you continue.
Grade*	**Time to Implement** – It takes 60
Difficulty 6	days to start **feeling** results from
	meditation.
Time to Implement 60 Days	**Importance** – Meditation can help
Importance 9	**every** aspect of wellness in a
*Amount is based off of the average person. Your personal results may be higher or lower depending on your specific needs.	multitude of ways.

18

The mental edge

Have you ever heard the saying, "It's all in your head?" Well, it most certainly is! If you can't get your head straight, how will you be able to achieve goals when it comes to health and fat loss? Think about it, where does the stress, tension, fatigue and negative thoughts that we play in our heads daily actually come from? It's all in our heads, meaning our subconscious or conscious thoughts. That's why meditation will be one of the most important recommendations in this book. When you start to control your thoughts, you'll have more willpower, less stress, more energy and/ or enhance your quality of sleep. In reality, there is nothing that you can't get BETTER at.

What do you think the first step of changing is? You guessed it, creating awareness about **how** you are thinking. How can you change anything if you're not constantly aware that you need to change? Also, how can you change if you don't put your energy toward a specific response?

Karl Moore, creator of the ZEN12 meditation program, explained, "The benefits of meditation are astonishing. Over 3,000 scientific studies at independent universities and research institutes since 1970 have studied this phenomenon, with staggering results."[2]

Jonathan Haidts book, *The Happiness Hypothesis*, reveals the answer. He states, "Suppose you read about a pill that you could take once a day to reduce anxiety and increase your contentment. Would you take it? Suppose further that the pill has a great variety of side effects, all of them good: increased self-esteem, empathy, and trust; it even improves memory. Suppose, finally, that the pill is all natural and costs nothing. Now would you take it? The pill exists. It's called meditation."[1]

WHY ISN'T IT POPULAR?

So why is meditation not taught in grade school? Also, why isn't everyone spending the small amount of time and energy it takes to become good at meditation? The first reason is that it's not "packaged" and "sold" as a product. Therefore, who is making money off of it? Another unfortunate reason is that there is a negative dogma that you have to be some sort of hippie wearing a robe, sitting in a field to meditate. This is most definitely false!

CLEAR YOUR MIND

For thousands of years people of all religious and philosophical points of view have practiced meditation, including most world leaders. Meditation's primary side effect is becoming more present and aware in every one of our daily reactions. It's this clear thinking that helps us to be **less** judgmental and reactive and **more** compassionate and calm so that we can perform powerfully in life. Through this heightened awareness, we have the ability to disengage from our strong attachments to negative thoughts and beliefs, which we have been exposed to throughout our lives. For example, it might be perfectly normal for you to unwind from a stressful day with a couple of glasses of wine because your parents did the same thing. Not only is that unhealthy, but it will also NOT help you to reach your goals of becoming a better you! Suddenly, we realize that this was something that was implanted in our subconscious as children. Now that we are **aware** of this problem, we can **change** it.

Bill Harris explains in his book, *Thresholds of the Mind*, that the brain is divided into two hemispheres. The problem is that the mind has a built in duality, which causes a type of communication problem, brain lateralization, which forces you to see the world as two separate unities. The more one-sided a person's brain is, the more issues they have. The issues include feelings of fear, anxiety, separation, isolation and addiction. Bill notes that long-term studies indicate that meditation actually balances the brain[3]!

INCREASE WILLPOWER

In the book, *The Willpower Instinct*, Kelly McGonigals explains you will receive heightened willpower from meditation, which in turn increases your odds for success in life. Willpower – not intelligence – is the blueprint for being extremely successful! Willpower outperforms IQ by a factor of two. She states, "Neuroscientists have discovered that when you ask the brain to meditate, it gets better not just at meditating, but at a wide range of self-control skills, including attention, focus, stress management, impulse control, and people who meditate regularly aren't just better at these things. Over time, their brains become finely tuned willpower machines. Regular meditators have more gray matter in the prefrontal cortex, as well as regions of the brain that support self-awareness[4]."

*Gray matter: The section of the brain involved in learning and memory procedures, emotional directive, self-referential managing and perspective taking[5]

Still not sold? Take the 8-week study on meditation where participants meditated for 12 to 15 minutes daily, which revealed that meditation actually changed the genetic expression in 2,209 genes[6]! Therefore, meditation has even crossed over into what was called the human genome project. This study is the forefront of what we know as "epigenetics." This just means that we all have a genetic disposition, but you can positively or negatively change the way that your genetics reacts to your environment. This just proves that meditation enhances all the good!

STRENGTHEN STRESS MANAGEMENT

Meditation is also critical for stress management as it allows us to get out of the "stew" of the modern day stresses. When you are stressed (AKA in fight or flight mode), your blood goes to your extremities rather than to your brain and digestive system. When your digestive system, the main passage to health and immunity, is compromised in this way, unfriendly toxins can enter your body and lead to disease. Additionally, when your blood is drawn away from your brain while stressed, thinking becomes harder. So using meditation to get out of a stressed state will allow us to think clearly and increase the proficiency of our immune system!

Even ABC news reported, "Several studies suggest that changes through meditation can make you happier, less stressed-even nicer to other people. It can help you control eating habits and even reduce chronic pain, all the while without taking prescription medications."

Last time I checked, being happy is priceless.

There are SO many ways to meditate, but let's start slow and simple.

STEP 1: "GOT PURPOSE?" FIND YOUR PERSONAL REASON TO MEDITATE

Having my Master's Degree in Applied Clinical Nutrition, being an ACE Certified Personal Trainer, Health Coach and former paramedic, my personal purpose is that I want to make a difference in people's lives. In order to do that, I have to be very intelligent and productive. During my tenure as a paramedic, the most gratifying part of my job was to help people. During the simple discharges from a hospital to a nursing home with an extremely scared dementia patient, I eased the patient's anxiety by introducing them to all the staff instead of dropping them off and running out the door. Over time, my purpose expanded because I have dyslexia and have struggled academically my entire life. Meditation and wellness improved – nearly to the point of reversing – my dyslexia and other problems that I had been struggling with previously. This is why taking the time to find your purpose is so important.

STEP 2: "SHOWING UP" IS 80% OF SUCCESS

Daily practice breeds success! Notice I didn't say four or six times a week. Do it EVERY DAY no matter what! If you give yourself wiggle room, your practice could fall off, so make it a daily routine! This will help ensure success. Start slow with 1-5 minutes, and then see what works specifically for you! Even if it's one minute daily, just get it in. It took me six months to find my way, and it was worth it.

STEP 3: "SIT COMFORTABLE"

Make sure that you sit comfortably, but in an alert position with an upright spine. Once you sit up, roll your shoulders back and sit in a chair, on your knees, cross your legs, or whatever works best for you! The point is to sit with pride and not slouched over.

STEP 4: "STOP & SET YOUR PERSONAL INTENTION"

Prior to mediating I set my personal intention by telling myself, "I am going to enjoy this peace and quiet while stilling my mind and calming my thoughts." Then I find a quiet place to start. You can set an alarm on your phone for your time preference or download a guided meditation from the app store on your electronic device.

STEP 5: "OBSERVE WITHOUT STRESS"

Place your attention on your posture, feel the sense of grounding and balance, all while breathing naturally. Just allow your thoughts to unfold without stressing about it.

STEP 6: "HELP THE RUN-AWAY BRAIN & PLACING THE STAKE"

A common misconception is that people think their brain will shut off and become completely silent while meditating. Even the most experienced meditators have their brains wander. It's common for fantasy, daydreaming or compulsive thought to let your brain wander off. How do we change this? Let's use the analogy of hammering stakes in the ground to put up a tent. With time, the stakes will loosen, so just put them back in. Placing your stake is what you do with the wandering thoughts. Examples of your stake are observing your breaths flowing in and out naturally, counting your breaths from 10 to zero, listening to a guided meditation and saying a prayer or mantra. The most important part is to notice the wandering and fix it, because you don't want to waste your time daydreaming. AGAIN, it's creating awareness!

STEP 7: PLAYS OFF STEP SIX, "NO WORRIES"

Don't get stressed out when your stake becomes loose. Just say "No worries," and reclaim that stake. Now you have created awareness without any stress!

STEP 8: "FIND ONE AND STICK TO IT"

I see it all the time with people getting sucked into the "law of distraction," trying every meditation practice out there, and never ending up using one long enough to see the results. The most popular types of meditation include mindfulness meditation and transcendental meditation. Some popular teachers include Ram Dass, Eckhart Tolle, Ken Wilber, and John Main.

STEP 9: "DO YOU"

When I started my meditation journey, it took me months to get in a routine. I was only able to perform at a higher level when I put in time and effort consistently. The amount of time and effort will vary from person to person – we're all coming from different backgrounds with different skill sets. So if you can only handle a minute daily, then a minute is better than nothing! Concentrate on what you are capable of and within a few weeks you WILL progress. Do what you are able to do every day!

STEP 10: "ACTION"

Note that research shows you only need 12-15 minutes of meditation each day, so take some action on fitting this small time commitment into your life. You'll never see results without taking action! As Mahatma Gandhi famously said, "Be the change that you wish to see in the world." And that applies to the change that you wish to see in yourself as well! So if you want to change the way you think, increase your likelihood for success in any area of your life, become happier, pump up your brain and just have a better quality of life, give meditation a try.

*The Rant: Meditation has almost endless benefits when practiced daily for an extended period of time. I highly recommend you start and stick with meditation once you find your favorite form.

Lifestyle Scale	DESCRIPTION
Serving Size 1 Person Makes 1 Lifetime Result	**Difficulty** – With **distractions** all around us, getting a **quality** night of sleep is difficult.
Grade Per Person	
Grade	
Grade*	**Time to Implement** – It takes 21 days to **create** or **replace** a habit.
Difficulty 4	
Time to Implement 21 Days	**Importance** – Quality sleep will result in more **energy**, which leads to **better** results.
Importance 7	
*Amount is based off of the average person. Your personal results may be higher or lower depending on your specific needs.	

19

Sleep hygiene

Are you one of those people who says, "I'll sleep when I'm dead," then walks around like a zombie all day? Sleep can be the missing link when it comes to both your health **and** happiness! Lack of sleep can be a major cause of the health problems throughout your life, including cancer.

Cancer? Really? Yes. The Center for Disease Control and Prevention reported that shift work, which causes a lack of sleep, is a known carcinogen[1]. The World Health Organization International Agency for Research on Cancer classified shift work as a "probable" carcinogen[2]. The U.S. Institute of Medicine's committee on sleep noted that after decades of research, they determined that a lack of sleep is associated with a wide range of detrimental health concerns that include an increased risk of hypertension, diabetes, obesity, depression, heart attack and stroke[3]. Equally troubling is that the National Sleep Foundation[4] found that over 50% of Americans are sleep deprived, and CNN interactive has reported sleep deprivation as the #1 health problem facing Americans today[5].

BETTER SLEEP = BETTER LIFE

So it's pretty simple: the better you sleep, the higher-quality life you will have! Because without sleep, whatever diseases or medical conditions you have or are at risk for having, will get worse. Now this research doesn't just mean you should sleep your life away. Oversleeping – just like overeating and over-training – creates its own health risks. So as we have with foods, let's increase the **quality** of your sleep as opposed to the **quantity**!

Several published studies concluded that poor sleep is a major risk factor of weight gain. Just one night of inadequate sleep can dramatically increase your food appetite and make you as insulin-resistant as a type II diabetic[6, 7].

The increase in appetite happens from hormonal imbalances. The hunger hormone (ghrelin) dramatically increases, causing you to feel extremely hungry. Then leptin, the hormone that tells your brain you aren't hungry anymore, takes a leave of absence!

The insulin resistance happens because of a lack of sleep causes your body to experience changes in its carbohydrate metabolism, hormone levels, autonomic nervous system activity and much more, including insulin malfunction when it's released into your blood stream[8]. Insulin-resistance causes chronically high insulin levels within the body, which leads to elevated blood sugar levels. Elevated blood sugar levels cause proteins and carbohydrates to combine, forming advanced glycation end-products or AGEs. AGEs increase cortisol, which destabilizes protein collagen and increases stress, which leads to premature aging of your skin and organs. Yikes!

The cycle of insulin resistance then goes like this: you eat food, which causes you to make insulin, which transports nutrition from the food you eat to either be stored as fat or to your muscles to be used for immediate energy. Since insulin is a transporting hormone, and insulin is malfunctioning, your body will **not** place this energy into your cells. When this resistance of insulin happens, the body cannot use the food for energy, which leaves you feeling tired and hungry while your body stores this energy as fat! Double whammy!

Most of us lead busy lives, which usually translates to grabbing some caffeine, sugar, or both to power through those long, tired hours until the end of the day. With prolonged use, caffeine can down-regulate your adrenal glands (you can only squeeze so much energy out of them), making any type of insulin resistance and hormonal imbalances even worse! Note that sugar is the main dietary culprit for causing insulin resistance. Nancy Appleton, PhD, devoted her life to explaining how sugar is a poison, and how it's actually as addictive as heroin!

KNOW YOUR SLEEP HORMONES

The hormone that most affects your ability to sleep is melatonin, which is made in your pineal gland. To understand how to effectively utilize your melatonin levels it's important to understand another hormone, serotonin, which some people call the "happy hormone."

Serotonin and melatonin work in total opposition, meaning that when serotonin is elevated, melatonin is repressed. You need high melatonin and low serotonin at night so that you can sleep. The opposite goes for the daytime. You should have high serotonin and low melatonin levels during the day for you to be energetic, alert and happy all day.

When you keep these hormones in check, sleep becomes easier, leading you to be healthier and happier. Light levels, certain medications, ingesting high amounts of carbs (especially late at night) and cell-phone use (which inhibits the pineal gland's ability to produce melatonin due to micro-wave-like frequencies) could be sabotaging your melatonin levels. Serotonin can also be sabotaged by being exposed to poor lighting all day and not getting out in the sun.

*There are so many tips that can aid you when trying to improve your sleep quality, but implementing only one probably won't help. If you are a life-long bad sleeper I highly recommend that you implement all of them and in time they will make a major difference!

FIND YOUR HIDDEN STRESSORS

You might not think so, but stressors in your life, whether obvious or hidden, can be the reason you are constantly kept up at night! For example smart phones, TVs, mobile devices and computers are a fairly new form of life-consuming unconscious stress that our bodies are not used to. This all adds up to unconscious stress, which people are actually unable to unplug from – even after turning off the screens and closing our eyes! The human brain is not meant to be "on" all the time. This causes an overload of sensory stimulation, increasing stress and decreasing sleep!

*Unconscious stress: A form of stress that stimulates the release of cortisol.

There's going to be a lot of factors that are simply out of our control when it comes to improving sleep quality, like being called into work or tending to loved ones in the middle of the night. But we're not here for doom and gloom, so let's focus on what we CAN control. Good sleep isn't something that just happens, so you'll need to put in a little attention and effort!

SLEEP IS CRITICAL

Simply acknowledging that sleep is critical and creating an awareness of this is the first crucial step in the process. During the day, be sure to get outside and soak up some natural rays, which lets your body produce serotonin, the happy hormone, which effectively stores your melatonin until the sun goes down and you're ready to sleep. Exercising is also crucial as physical activity actually flushes out stress hormones like cortisol from your body. You should be careful not to perform any high-intensity exercises two hours prior to bedtime if you are having trouble sleeping because endorphins and other chemicals that are released into your bloodstream during exercise make you more energetic and alert, which is obviously counterproductive to getting a restful night's sleep. Light exercise at night like taking a walk around the neighborhood, however, can help you to unwind and further promote your quality of sleep.

CAFFEINE, ALCOHOL & NICOTINE - OH MY!

Sleep experts stress caffeine – found mostly in coffee, tea, soda and chocolate – should not be ingested after 3:00 p.m. because it takes 12 hours to fully metabolize caffeine's effects throughout the body. So if you drink caffeine at 3:00 p.m., you'll still have half of that caffeine in your blood stream at 9:00 p.m. Remember that "decaf" DOESN'T necessarily mean "no caffeine!" The Journal of Analytical Toxicology examined nine different decaffeinated coffees, and eight of them had 8.6 to 13.9 mg of caffeine[9].

*Even though regular coffee has much more caffeine (around 95mg), 8.6 to 13.9mg is enough to cause sleep issues.

Alcohol is the most commonly abused substance in the world and is NOT advisable to help you sleep! While at first it acts as a depressant, it becomes a stimulant after several hours, at which point it can then interfere with the quality of your sleep and wake you up in the middle of the night. And even though some of you might not wake up, alcohol **will** disturb your mind throughout the night, causing a lower quality and restless sleep.

Nicotine should also be avoided because it's a central nervous system stimulant. People think it's calming them down when in reality it's only satisfying their withdrawal symptoms.

UNWIND THE MIND

Meditation is a great relaxation technique that creates awareness in your life, helps control a racing mind and releases the day's stresses and tensions in order to allow you to sleep properly. You can also write down a task list for the next day before bed, which will help to clear your late-night mind of anxieties.

Unwinding prior to bed is critical when it comes to sleep hygiene. Do these by establishing bedtime rituals like pleasurable reading, drinking a small cup of night-time tea, unplugging from technology, using a candle for light or performing a relaxation breathing technique.

You can use this relaxing breathing technique that is recommended by sleep experts:

- Place the tip of your tongue against the ridge behind your front teeth and exhale completely through your mouth.
- Inhale through your nose to a count of four.
- Hold your breath to a count of seven.
- Exhale through your mouth with a swooshing sound to the count of eight.
- Repeat this cycle for a total of four breaths prior to bedtime and you'll notice the difference in your stress levels.

FIGHT YOUR SLEEP ROBBERS

There are several common "sleep robbers" that could be affecting you.

The most common are:

- Noise
- Light

- Room temperature
- TV
- Computers
- Sleep partners
- Pets

Let's actually take a closer look into these. We should be sleeping 1/3 of each 24-hour period (that's eight hours), so spending money on a good mattress, pillows and sheets are sound investments! A white-noise machine or fan leaves your brain at a constant signal so other little noises don't wake you up. Your room should be extremely dark, and a temperature of 65 to 72 degrees will keep your body in a thermally neutral state. Eliminate noise distractions like locking the cat out of the bedroom if it's running across your bed every night, or wearing earplugs if your partner snores. Believe it or not, clutter in your bedroom can distract you from sleep too because it creates unconscious stress!

There's a saying, "One hour before midnight is worth two after," which means that your best-quality sleep is obtained between 10 pm and 5 am, when the body is at its natural sleep cycle. If you have children, you know things become a mess once they are off their schedule, and the same goes for you! No matter how old you are, create a regular bedtime for yourself because the body loves repetition, predictability and pattern. If you work irregular shifts and/or sleep during the day, you should still make sure that you are going to sleep around the same time each day. A consistent bed time, even if less than ideal, will lead you to get to bed easier and faster!

TONE DOWN THE LIGHT

*Amber lighting is more soothing to the brain, which helps you to unwind prior to bedtime.

Reduce artificial light several hours prior to bed (candles work best as a more natural source of illumination after the sun goes down). This means no computer two hours prior to bed because of the high-intensity blue light that it gives off! The more "blue" the light, the higher the temperature on the Kelvin scale.

To give you a better understanding of the Kelvin scale, candle-light is measured at 1800 Kelvin, incandescent indoor lights are 3000 Kelvin, ultraviolet noon sunlight is 5500 Kelvin, and the light emitted from a computer screen is listed at 6500 Kelvin!

If you NEED to use your computer at night, try the free downloadable program called f.Lux, which improves the quality of your sleep by removing the "blue light" from the screen at night. It also automatically adjusts the "blue light" to be higher during daylight hours!

ELIMINATE ELECTRONICS AT NIGHT

Stop talking on your cell phone after 6:00 p.m. without using wired earphones or the phone speaker for calls. Or just text. Whatever it takes to avoid putting the phone up to your face because the microwave-like frequencies from the constant information your phone is uploading and downloading will run through your brain and keep it stimulated at night. If you use your cell phone for an alarm, consider a basic alarm clock instead. You should turn off any other digital devices, including your wireless router - even if it's in a different room – as it can be interfering with your sleep!

Reduce the lighting in your bedroom by using blackout shades for your windows and turn your alarm clock around so the light isn't being cast directly onto you.

Keep your bed for sleeping and sex – that's it! Sleep experts explained that the bedroom is your sanctuary and you shouldn't watch TV, play on the computer or anything else for that matter.

*Ask your doctor or pharmacist if some natural sleep remedies are right for you. Just make sure that you do your own research too! Melatonin has a lot of research behind it, especially when used for correcting irregular sleep patterns (i.e. jet lag) and to counteract the side effects of medications that deplete melatonin levels as well as the inevitable loss of melatonin as you age. Like any supplement or medication, though, don't depend on them!

HOW MUCH SLEEP DO WE NEED?
You should be aiming for 7-8 hours of sleep each night, but everyone is different, so if you do well with a little more or less, then do what works for you!

I know that some of these tips may be extremely hard to do if these habits have been part of your life for such a long time, but not only will you feel more energetic and alert, but it'll help you lose unwanted body fat even faster.

*The Rant: Without proper sleep, your body will experience multiple negative side effects such as hormonal imbalances, decreased energy, insulin malfunction and much more!

Lifestyle Scale	DESCRIPTION
Serving Size 1 Person Makes 1 Lifetime Result	**Difficulty** – Stress is very difficult to **manage,** but gets easier with time.
Grade Per Person	
Grade	
Grade*	**Time to Implement** – Stress will **always** be a part of your life.
Difficulty 9	
Time to Implement Never Ending	**Importance** – Managing stress will help you **stay healthy** from the inside-out.
Importance 8	
*Amount is based off of the average person. Your personal results may be higher or lower depending on your specific needs.	

20

Stress management

Stress is the inability to cope with a threat to your well-being, whether it is real or imagined, and results in a series of responses and adaptations by your body in order to protect itself. Stress affects your mind, body, emotions and behaviors because your body thinks that it's being threatened in some way, like being chased by a lion, when, in reality, a coworker just pissed you off. If you can't learn how to control this stress, you will not be able to lose weight permanently!

The latest estimates revealed that 75-90% of physician's office appointments were for symptoms that were stress related[1]. This just goes to show that stress is a big problem!

Managing stress is so difficult because it requires us to change core patterns of belief and behavior, which is in itself, extremely stressful! What you need to know is that keeping this feeling of worry, fear and anxiousness in check will lead to advances in almost every aspect of your life. No matter how you look at it, stress management is critical to your overall health, and if you don't have your health, what's really left?

WIRED TO THINK NEGATIVELY

As humans, we are automatically wired to attract negative thoughts instead of positive ones. Think about it, most people are more willing to go online and write a bad review of a restaurant before they would ever be willing to write a positive one. Sad but true.

Dr. Hanson states that, "Our ancestors could make two kinds of mistakes, 1. Thinking there was a tiger in the bushes when there wasn't one, and 2. Thinking there was no tiger in the bushes when there actually was one. The cost of the first mistake was needless stress, while the cost of the second one was death. Consequently, we evolved to make the first mistake a thousand times to avoid making the second mistake even once."[2] Rewiring our brain to think in the positive is a hard but POSSIBLE task that just takes time.

STRESS AND YOUR FITNESS

Stress can single-handedly destroy any attempts when trying to achieve a fitness goal. This is why I would really like for you to tune in on reducing stress as much as possible. You can have the best diet, the hardest workouts, take the most expensive supplements on the market, and stress can actually negate them all! Learning how to control stress is not only going to help you be **healthier**, but it's also going to make you **happier**.

Chronic stress is a real killer, and it gets worse with time if not managed! Cortisol is a hormone most commonly associated with stress, which is released in a specific rhythm throughout the day to keep you energetic and alert by activating your adrenal glands. Normally cortisol is high in the morning to help you wake up and go about your day, and low in the evening to help you get to sleep. However, stress breaks this rhythm by stopping cortisol from being released in the morning and increasing the levels released in the evening, causing inflammation, deprived sleep and serious weight gain.

Chronic stress, prolonged stress or worrying tells the body to produce cortisol, and when cortisol is elevated, it marks a decrease in leptin, your hunger hormone that lets you know when you should stop eating[3]. So a decrease in leptin increases your hunger, which leads to overeating. Now, a combination of decreased leptin and elevated cortisol will lower your metabolism in the long-run, causing massive fat storage. Adding insult to injury, your body stores this fat especially around the mid-section because it's close to your intestines and your brain thinks that you are being at-tacked all the time, so it places the fat in an easily accessible spot.

When weight is stored in your stomach, it's called having an "apple-shaped body," in contrast to a having a "pear-shaped body," where fat is stored in your hips and thighs. People with an apple-shaped body are at more risk for health problems associated with obesity like coronary heart disease, high blood pressure and diabetes[4].

SOME FOOD CAUSES STRESS!

What you consume, and when you consume it, cannot only affect your body, but it can also affect your mind! The overconsumption of caffeinated beverages such as coffee or energy drinks can fatigue our adrenal glands, thereby causing stress. Chronic inflammation throughout the body can also be a huge part of why our brain is feeling so stressed throughout the day. Cleaning up your diet cannot only detoxify your body, but it can also do the same for your mind. Ingesting anti-inflammatory foods such as green veggies, avocados, berries and fatty fish can help reduce this inflam-mation and lead to lower levels of stress in your body.

Because stress burns through essential vitamins and minerals, it is a major contributor to fatigue, nutrient depletion and micronutrient deficiencies within the body. The combination of a poor diet and chronic stress makes nutrient depletion even more severe because of the "empty calories" that any processed and fast foods give your body. Making matters worse, your body uses nutrients to process these processed and fast foods, so the negative effects are accelerated!

Magnesium is an essential mineral that's involved in over 300 biochemical reactions in your body, including aiding in the functions for energy, metabolism, muscle contraction, vasodilation of the coronary and peripheral arteries, nerve depolarization and benefits to bone and tooth health[5]. Deficiencies in magnesium are correlated with eye disease, heart disease, increased insulin sensitivity and an increase in blood pressure. Believe it or not, that is just a deficiency from **one** mineral.

ANXIETY IS STRESS

Anxiety is another form of stress that you must learn to control. There is a difference between fear and anxiety. Fear is a feeling that we get when there is a threat to ourselves. Anxiety is a worry about the possibilities that could go wrong in the future. To help control this feeling you should "live in the now." By "living in the now," you can tell yourself that everything is fine and suppress that feeling of worry about the future.

CHALLENGE YOURSELF

Unlike stress, a challenge is an important ingredient for healthy and productive work. However, a challenge is often confused as stress when, in reality, it energizes individuals both psychologically and physically. It motivates people to learn new skills, master their jobs, and when a challenge is met, people feel relaxed and satisfied.

STARTING STRESS MANAGEMENT

So now that you're familiar with the problems associated with uncontrolled stress, how are you going to start stress management? There are so many methods and techniques to explore, but let's look at just a few so as not to overwhelm and stress you since that's exactly the opposite of what we're trying to do here.

A good start is to create awareness about where your stress is coming from! Taking a step back from your hectic life and taking 10 deep breaths slowly is a great way to slow down your world and clear your mind. Of course, finding sensible and meaningful ways to eliminate or at least reduce the stress from your life is the ultimate end game!

"Our life is shaped by our mind; we become what we think." - Buddha.

THERE'S ONLY 24 HOURS IN A DAY

You may be tempted to take on more than you can reasonably handle in your life. The truth is that there are only 24 hours a day, and only 16 left after sleeping. We all also have other obligations such as eating, working, spending time with family, working out, pursuing personal pleasures and the list goes on. It is important to "know thyself." That is, to know your stress limits and to know what's important to you and to your health. So make a goal of controlling your time. Prioritize what you need and figure out ways to cut back on what you don't need. It might be something as easy as using better communication skills by acknowledging what someone says by repeating it back to them. This is an effective technique because it shows the people around you that they are important because you are actively listening. And if the people around you feel like you value them, they are more likely to be working with you rather than against you, which means a whole lot less stress!

Lowering stressful experiences by learning to say no is one of the easiest ways to get rid of unnecessary stress. Don't take on more than you know you can handle, and avoid the people that stress you out in life. We all have some friends who are always taking and never giving, which might be a major cause of some of your stress. Turn off the news, or minimize the time you spend watching it, especially in the morning or before bed. The negativity will only wear on your conscience throughout the day and night. Give up on all pointless arguments that never seem to lead to any change. This could be with a spouse, friend or coworker. It could also be a specific topic of conversation such as politics or religion. If this is the case, then save yourself the trouble and don't even bring it up in conversation. Developing empathy by trying to understand other people's feelings will also help you understand your own. Practicing spirituality leads to less stress and a happier life.

MEDITATE YOUR MIND

Meditation has been proven to reduce stress in both the mind and body. Believe it or not, meditation can also help you torch body fat by reducing chronic stress and its negative health effects. A study conducted by the Cedars-Sinai Medical Center in Los Angeles concluded that Transcendental Meditation is proven to reduce hypertension, obesity and diabetes in patients with coronary heart disease. The study was conducted on 103 individuals with coronary heart disease. It found that these participants taking part in Transcendental Meditation for four months had lower blood pressure, improved blood glucose, improved insulin levels and a more stable function of their autonomic nervous system.

REWIRE YOUR BRAIN

Turn your negative thoughts into positive ones by finding the silver lining. Marketing agencies, news outlets, and political spokespersons do this all the time – they take something bad and "spin" it so that you see the good in it. For instance, if you've "only" lost an inch off your waistline, don't think of it as having "only" lost an inch – instead, think of it as being one inch closer to your ideal waistline. Take this positive thought and repeat it over and over in your head until you are able to believe in it. Meditation is a great way to create awareness in this sort of situation, so don't be afraid to use it.

Look at bad situations as a time for personal growth. Making it through the hard times only makes the good times even better. Major challenges will always face us, but taking the bull by the horns and defeating these challenges leads you to be a better, stronger you!

Some great ways to practice your relaxation skills are through meditation, tai chi, yoga, drinking hot tea, deep breathing techniques, chi gong, progressive muscular relaxation, musical therapy, exercising or even loving someone. Doing something as simple as hugging a loved one can calm your body by decreasing your cortisol levels. Of course, there's also pursuing a hobby, participating in a social group, or just taking the time to laugh at some good old fashioned comic relief.

ONLY BRING POSITIVE ENERGY

Try to go easy with criticism, because even though you might be trying to help, criticism brings negative energy! You only have so much energy, and when you create positive thoughts such as love and gratitude, you feel that positive energy. Be realistic in what you **can** accomplish compared to what you **would like** to accomplish. Failing to reach your goal zaps your willpower, so be sensible with your goals. FYI, willpower can be built through meditation. Anyway, if someone wants to lose 100 pounds in a few weeks, that's not only unrealistic, but it can be extremely detrimental to your health. Either way it will be a lose-lose, so instead set yourself up for goals that you can handle without selling yourself short.

*Meditation can help with treating unresolved anger or fear within your subconscious.

Make yourself aware of unresolved anger or fear that can be buried deep within your subconscious. If untreated, this unresolved stress will continue to tear you down from the inside out. There are several ways to resolve stress, but don't say I didn't warn you, because none are easy. In addition, all of them take a lot of time and willpower. Remember, hanging onto anger doesn't hurt the other person behind you, but it most certainly hurts you!

Because stress is a normal and natural hormonal response for when we are being chased by a lion, for example, exercise is a great way to naturally work stress out of the body as well as prevent its build up. Making time in your schedule for at LEAST 30 minutes of exercise a day will make a huge difference in how you feel, act and think. Even so, you still need to be careful not to overtrain as doing so will create stress on your body! Most people are not professional athletes or Olympians, so it's important to let our bodies rest after training intensely. Constant stress with no rest will work against your body and actually cause negative effects. This is usually prevalent in people who train 6-7 days a week with no "rest day." Setting aside this relaxation time gives you a break from all the worry in your life.

FLUSH YOUR STRESS THROUGH WRITING

Keeping a "stress journal" where all of your fears and anxieties can live without causing any sort of stress can stop you from feeling overwhelmed. And with so many people to see and activities to accomplish, the journal can also help you prioritize what is important in your life in addition to clearing up all the mixed thoughts in your head. A time management calendar, whether an app on your phone or physical, will also help to eliminate anxieties.

DO WHAT YOU CAN CONTROL

Make sure that your create awareness around what you CAN control. Try to let go of the negativity of what you CAN'T control. If you know that the grocery store is going to be packed today, but you know it will be a ghost town tomorrow, WAIT! If you know your commute home will be lined with traffic, but there is an alternative route that is clear from traffic, take the less stressful way. Even if it takes you a couple of minutes longer, the relief from the stress of a packed road will be worth it. Since you have no control over your environment, take control of your actions that you take in that environment.

THE POWER OF GRATITUDE

Using the power of gratitude will help ease the pressure and stress of life. Writing down five things that you are grateful for in your "Gratitude Journal" is a proven way to lower stress and increase happiness. Whether it's your family, job, house or pet, there is always something that you can be grateful for each day. The trick is to always find something different to be grateful for daily!

Even though we all love to get our way all the time, it's not a reality! Therefore, being able to compromise is a great tool that will reduce stress and help you to get further in life with other people. Now that doesn't mean that you should bend over backward for everyone in every situation, but getting "an even piece of the pie" will help you to feel satisfied. Dealing with your problems directly will help resolve any unconscious stress that could be lingering in the back of your mind. Taking an assertive call to action will help lead you to solutions, but doing it in a respectful way still remains extremely important!

NEW FORMS OF STRESS

Smartphones, TVs, mobile devices and computers are a fairly new form of stress that our bodies aren't used to. The constant stimulation from these devices is unnatural and creates unconscious stress. Instead of using these devices, turn them off and find something to do outside that you enjoy. Take the dog for a walk, play with the kids or go sightseeing. The energy that you will gain from getting out in the sun and in nature will help decrease any stress hormones in your body.

*The Rant: Even with the most intense workout regimen, the best nutrition plan and the most willpower to succeed, stress can single-handedly destroy all of your attempts. Therefore, managing this stress will accelerate progress in every other aspect of health.

Lifestyle Scale	DESCRIPTION
Serving Size 1 Person Makes 1 Lifetime Result	**Difficulty** – With so much **negativity** hardwired into our brains from evolution and society, it is difficult to stay **truly** happy.
Grade Per Person	
Grade	
Grade*	
Difficulty 8	**Time to Implement** – It takes 21 days to **create** or **replace** a habit.
Time to Implement 21 Days	**Importance** – Creating **happiness** will increase **willpower**.
Importance 7	
*Amount is based off of the average person. Your personal results may be higher or lower depending on your specific needs.	

21

Happiness

Happiness is a mental or emotional state of well-being characterized by positive or pleasant emotions.

When you reduce stress and increase happiness, you'll feel better, have a more positive outlook on life, have more energy and increase your willpower, all of which will help you lose unwanted fat. When I say "happiness," I am referring to TRUE happiness in general. A lot of people are "happy" in certain aspects of their lives, whether it's financially, professionally or something else. **True** happiness leads to fulfillment in finances, career, personal relationships and more!

It has been shown that 60% of feeling happy is based on your personality, but the other 40% is completely modifiable from your personal thoughts and behaviors[1]. That's great news, because it means that you can make massive strides toward your well-being while increasing your happiness by changing the way you think and act!

Everyone has different criteria for happiness, so ignore the tips that don't work for you, but daily embrace and apply the tips that resonate with you. That's the only way to make a change in the amount of happiness you experience in your life.

SURROUND YOURSELF WITH HAPPINESS

One of the best ways to create happiness is to surround yourself with happy and loving people! Nurturing and strengthening relationships with friends or family takes time, and isn't everyone's strong point. Still, take a minute to be thankful for your life each day when you wake up and before you go to bed. I always emphasize being thankful for something new every day as this will truly create gratitude. It's better to be aware of the simple parts of your life that you're thankful for **now** and to express that gratitude **now** rather than putting it off until tragedy strikes and it's too late to say everything that you've been holding in. So instead be thankful for what you have each day starting now!

Performing random acts of kindness is the most dependable way of increasing your well-being, since they are both easy and effective. Go out and volunteer for something or give blood at a drive if you're eligible to. I can almost guarantee that you will get that warm feeling deep down. Cultivate optimism by working on seeing the positive aspects in your life. Know that what's right about you personally always trumps what's wrong! Thinking and speaking negatively will fill your body and mind with negative energy, so look to the people in your life that are filled with positive energy and find the inspiration in them to lead a more positive life. Laughter, misery, anxiety, fear and other emotions are all contagious, so be sure that you're surrounding yourself with people who keep a positive outlook on life.

YOUR PERCEPTION SHAPES YOUR WORLD

Sometimes things in life don't go as we hoped or planned, but your perception will shape how you respond. When the situations occur, take a step back to create awareness, then ask yourself, "Is there a different way that I can look at this?" and, "Is it really that bad of a situation?" Not only will this help you decipher the good, the bad and the ugly, but it will also give you a minute to process exactly what is going on so that you can respond in a healthy and appropriate way. And who knows? Maybe however the situation turned out isn't actually that big of a deal.

DO IT FOR YOURSELF

Be sure to take time for yourself so that you can find your true purpose for everything you do and want to do in your life. Thinking critically about and clearly identifying what you want out of life will help you manifest true happiness. How do you want to be remembered? What excites you? What makes you proud? These are all great questions that you can ask yourself in order to feel that sense of fulfillment in your life that truly means something to you.

As with everything, practice makes perfect! Your thoughts affect your behavior, and your behavior shapes your actions. So try hard every day and keep your thoughts positive.

*The Rant: By changing the way you think and act you will be able to increase your happiness immensely, which will lead to an increase in willpower!

Lifestyle Scale	DESCRIPTION
Serving Size 1 Person Makes 1 Lifetime Result	**Difficulty – Naturally** detoxifying is the hardest part.
Grade Per Person	
Grade	**Time to Implement** – It takes 14 days to **naturally** detoxify your body.
Grade*	
Difficulty 4	
Time to Implement 14 Days	**Importance** – Naturally detoxifying your body will **help** all other aspects of **permanent** fat loss.
Importance 6	
*Amount is based off of the average person. Your personal results may be higher or lower depending on your specific needs.	

22

How to: naturally detoxify

There is a ridiculous amount of so-called "Detoxification Programs" out there that are doing more harm than good. Misleading advertising, improper dosing of supplementation and even unsafe fasting can cause people to become more toxic than when they first started[1]. Therefore, you HAVE to realize what toxins you have been exposed to so that you can safely and effectively detoxify yourself[1].

WE ALL HAVE THEM
We all have small amounts of toxins in our body, so there is no need to panic, but when an excess of these toxins builds up and overwhelms our bodies – that's when disease sets in. Detoxification is not a single reaction, but rather an entire process that involves numerous reactions and multiple players.

"Detoxification is central to understanding functional assessment in medicine not so much because we live in a toxic environment, but because detoxification is the biggest item in everyone's biochemical budget. It handles waste not only from our environment, but from every process in all the organs and systems of the body." - Sidney Baker, MD[2]

THE LIVER IS CRUCIAL

The majority of detoxification takes place primarily in the liver, secondarily in the small intestines and finally in other tissues as well. The liver is really the most important detoxification point in the body though.

Your liver has two phases of detoxification. In the first phase, the liver takes the toxins and makes them more harmful than the original substance. In the second phase, the liver transforms these detrimental substances into easily excreted water-soluble compounds such as sweat and urine. If Phase 1 detoxification increases, which can happen when detox supplements are taken incorrectly, and Phase 2 detoxifications remain slow to normal, the body can actually become more toxic! This is the most important reason why you MUST be extremely cautious when using any detoxification supplements[1, 3].

PROPER MAKES PERMANENT

PROPER detoxification is also critical when it comes to PERMANENT weight loss because if you have a surplus of toxins in your bloodstream, your body's metabolism will slow down[4]. Your body tells your thyroid to stop working, immediately storing the toxins as fat cells so that your body doesn't get overwhelmed. Eating **quality** foods will reduce the amount of toxins you're putting into your body, which translates into losing fat faster. Eating quality, organic, local foods will also allow your body to release more body fat, and who doesn't want that?

WHAT ABOUT FASTING?

Some people fast in order to increase detoxification, and while it can work for **some** people, most often it does more harm than good. Fasting increases your Phase 1 detoxification, making you more toxic;

it decreases antioxidants, which then stresses all of your bodily functions, and the lack of dietary nutrition can also impair Phase 2 of your liver detoxification[1, 3]. Additionally, you won't be able to eliminate your waste when you don't eat dietary fibers, which can kill off your healthy gut bacteria!

MAKE THE CHANGES

So, instead of going on some extreme, non-sustainable, lifestyle altering detoxification diet, make the PROPER lifestyle changes so that you are always detoxifying your body naturally.

It's easier than you might think.

- Drink plenty of filtered water: 9 glasses for women and 13 glasses for men per day.
- Move your bowels at least 2-3 times per day. If this is a problem increase your fiber and healthy fat intake using two tablespoons of fresh ground flaxseed. Make sure you are getting enough water, as outlined above, and use a quality probiotic as well.
- Eat 10-12 servings of mainly vegetables and small amount of fruit daily. Eat the full rainbow of colors in vegetables.
- Eat vegetables that are high in sulfur like collards, cabbage, Brussel sprouts, broccoli, kale, onions and garlic.
- Eliminate or greatly reduce any alcohol intake.
- Eliminate or extremely reduce stimulants like caffeine or nicotine.
- Eliminate all sugar and flour.
- Sweat profusely daily, or at least three times per week using, for example, a steam room or sauna, or wear extra layers while working out. Remember to hydrate properly with water immediately after and to replace your electrolytes with a quality salt in your next meal.
- Exercise at high levels of intensity (only after being cleared by your doctor for the activity, of course).
- Take high-quality vitamins and minerals.

*Quality salt: Look for a sea salt or Himalayan salt with only one ingredient on the label.

Finally, use stress-reduction techniques, get some quality sleep and move more each day!

*The Rant: Detoxifying naturally will bring your body better and longer-lasting results. Do not fall victim to these quick fix "detoxifying programs."

Lifestyle Scale	DESCRIPTION
Serving Size 1 Person Makes 1 Lifetime Result	**Difficulty** – Finding **quality** supplements is the hardest part.
Grade Per Person	
Grade	
Grade*	**Time to Implement** – It takes 21 days to **create** or **replace** a habit.
Difficulty 2	
Time to Implement 21 Days	**Importance** – If **deficient**, adding these supplements will aid in **permanent** fat loss.
Importance 7	
*Amount is based off of the average person. Your personal results may be higher or lower depending on your specific needs.	

23

Supplements – do we need them?

The truth is that CERTAIN supplements definitely have a place in our diet because of the low-quality foods that surround us almost everywhere we go! Foods that are really old, picked prior to being ripe and are extremely processed are all lacking the proper nutrition that your body truly needs because anytime food is removed from its natural state its quality degrades. This is all too common because many food manufacturers are making food as cheaply as possible, which results in the lowest quality food they can possibly offer that people will still buy! For example, in the movie "The Healing Effect," Jan Zeff explained that 1 cup of spinach from 1945 equals 65 cups of spinach's nutritional value today. Not only that, but there are 1,200 additives in some current food supplies, which further increases the need for micronutrients and proper detoxification[1].

MICRONUTRIENTS MATTER

Micronutrients play an important role in how your body reacts to different types of foods. There have been numerous studies which show the correlation that deficiencies in vitamins, minerals and vitamin-like substances have been directly linked to weight gain and obesity.

Jayson Calton, PhD, published the results of a study he conducted in the journal *Economics and Human Biology*[2]. In it, his results showed that participants had an 80.8% higher chance of being overweight or obese **due to** micronutrient deficiencies compared to those who were not micronutrient deficient.

- Potassium Deficiency – 9 out of 10 Americans
- Vitamin E Deficiency – 8 out of 10 Americans
- Vitamin A Deficiency – 7 out of 10 Americans
- Vitamin C Deficiency – 7 out of 10 Americans
- Magnesium Deficiency – 7 out of 10 Americans

These deficiencies are coming from Americans who are eating "empty calories," but also people who are trying to lose weight improperly and unhealthily. So eating fake foods and meal replacements will definitely create certain vitamin and mineral deficiencies when true whole food sources are cut out of the diet.

SUPPLEMENT A PROPER NUTRITION PLAN

Prior to beginning any supplement regimen, you should always have a sound nutrition plan in place! Furthermore, never ingest a mega dose of vitamins because many vitamins and minerals fight for absorption in your intestines. This means that even though these massive amounts of vitamins and minerals are going in your mouth, they aren't actually being absorbed and utilized by your body. You only need a few supplements to give your body what it truly needs, and they have to be a **quality** product in order for them to work properly. **If you decide to take supplements, make sure to take a high-quality supplement from a trusted manufacturer or healthcare professional only, or don't take them at all!**

New regulatory requirements on dietary supplements DO NOT require FDA approval - or submission of efficacy and safety data - prior to marketing. The FDA's supplement division's own employees also explain that they are understaffed and under-funded! This means that we the tax payers have to show damage or submit a complaint before the process of removing the supplement from the market can even start.

MY RECOMMENDATIONS

The four supplements that I recommend are:

- an omega-3 fatty acid that contains EPA and DHA
- vitamin D3
- a probiotic
- a multi-vitamin mineral

Omega-3 fatty acids (EPA and DHA) are essential because humans are unable to synthesize them, so they must be obtained through your diet. The average American diet is at least 10-25 times higher in omega-6 fatty acids, which are inflammatory oils, compared to omega-3 fatty acids, which are anti-inflammatory oils[3]. This pro-inflammatory imbalance can lead to numerous health complications like inflammation, impaired cellular communication, a higher risk for cancer, auto-immune disease and cardiovascular disease just to name a few[4].

*EPA and DHA: Eicosapentaenoic acid (EPA) and docosahexaenoic acid (DHA) are two types of omega-3 fatty acids found in fatty fish.

With virtually all tissue throughout the body possessing a receptor for vitamin D3, this essential "vitamin" regulates almost 200 genes throughout the body, inhibits inflammation and actually boosts the immune system[5]! Although D3 is classified as a vitamin, it's actually a hormone that is made in the body when it absorbs energy from the sun! This means that if you are getting out in the sun during the day, you will probably not need to supplement D3. However, if you live in a climate or lead a particular lifestyle where you don't see the sun for an extended period of time, supplementing D3 is extremely important. I recommend that you get your levels tested in order to see where you stand!

Multi-vitamin minerals are the basic components of every cell within the body. They are essential to the body and most have limited storage. Marginal deficiencies are subtle and people tend not to be able to pinpoint why they feel off on any given day. These multi-vitamin minerals are important because of food refinement, processing and storage, which tend to strip foods of their original vitamin and mineral content. Think of a multi-vitamin mineral supplement as an insurance policy and take a high quality one in a low dose.

The final supplement that I recommend is a probiotic. Probiotics help build the "good bacteria" in your gastrointestinal (GI) tract, which protect your body from invaders and boost your digestive capabilities for the long-run. These are no different than any other supplement recommendation, the type and quality are what matter most! Make sure to ask your health care professional which is right for you. In addition, because probiotics are an emerging field, make sure to keep your eyes out for new research!

THE POINT

The main point that you should take from this is that ALL supplements work in CONJUNCTION with **proper nutrition**! Meals cannot be truly replaced with pills – but they can be supplemented.

*The Rant: As with your food, quality supplements can be extremely important in aiding you in your fat loss journey.

Lifestyle Scale	DESCRIPTION
Serving Size 1 Person Makes 1 Lifetime Result	**Difficulty – Repairing** previous **damage** is first and the hardest.
Grade Per Person	
Grade	**Time to Implement –** It takes 3 days to get in the **swing** of a **new** program.
Grade*	
Difficulty 4	**Importance –** Repairing **previous** fad diet damage it **crucial** in seeing lasting results.
Time to Implement 3 Days	
Importance 7	
*Amount is based off of the average person. Your personal results may be higher or lower depending on your specific needs.	

24

Fad diets

I really want to get the point across about how these fad diets are actually setting you back from your goals by damaging your metabolism and providing either a biased education or **no education** at all.

THEY SET YOU UP TO FAIL

Believe it or not, the diet industry as a whole has a 95% failure rate for consumers because the reality is that they are setting you up to fail because that's when you'll come back to them and buy more of their products[1]. Their business plan is simply to get you hooked for life. It's difficult to rake in BILLIONS of dollars if you're actually delivering real and true permanent weight loss, so it's in their best interests as a business, really.

FAKE FOODS AND MRPS

Really hot tickets on the market are these fake foods and meal replacement powders (MRPs). "Don't have time? Drink this powder!" "In a hurry? Eat this bar!" Well, the truth is that these processed, low-quality foods are missing naturally-occurring enzymes, phytonutrients, vitamins and minerals that real whole foods have in them and everything your body is looking for! These MRPs and fake foods are missing what's called the "sum of the whole food." For example, a tomato has a cancer fighting phytonutrient called lycopene in it. If you were to eat a whole tomato, you would receive its energy, information and lycopene. You might think that you can get away with just taking a lycopene pill, but your body will in fact notice the difference! And not having the "sum of the whole food" can cause more problems than solutions[2].

YOUR BRAIN KNOWS

When you ingest these fake foods, MRPs and pills, not only is your brain going to sense micronutrient deficiencies, but it will also sense that it's missing pleasure. This will cause your brain's hunger hormones like leptin, cholecystokinin, peptide YY and ghrelin to run ravenous and cause you to overeat. Your body is always looking for energy, information and nutrients, so if you aren't eating foods that are nutrient-rich, it's going to keep looking for them. Even if you are technically "full," your brain is going to tell you to keep eating away until it satisfies those **nutrient** needs.

WHY ARE YOU HUNGRY?

These are the top-six reasons why people are hungry in general, and especially on a diet:

1. Eating processed food-like substances
2. Lack of sleep
3. Micro and macro nutrient deficiencies
4. Dehydration
5. Lack of movement
6. Craving love and intimacy

THE FAD DIET WHEEL

Just like my Wellness Wheel, I have created something called a "Fad Diet Wheel," which is the total opposite of what you want when you are trying to get healthier. I call this the Fad Diet Wheel because it's a vicious circle that is never ending unless you are willing to stand up for yourself as a healthy and happy person to get out of it.

Check it out:

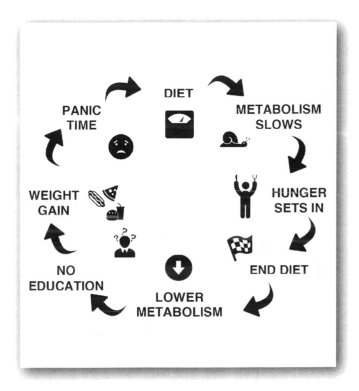

When you begin one of these fad diets, your metabolism is going to slow down, and then your hunger is going to set in from your hormones running ravenous because of your nutrient deficiencies. Maybe you'll see some results, but it's costing you the pleasure of eating real whole foods, and since you have been provided with a lowered metabolism and no education, you are very likely going to go back to your normal pre-diet eating habits. This leads to weight gain, and probably more than when you even started the diet in the first place. What's next? Panic time! You look for a new fad diet to go on, and the cycle starts all over again.

SKIP THE YO-YO DIETING

You have probably heard of this type of cycle referred to as the "yo-yo dieting effect," which is temporary weight loss followed by massive weight gain. A huge problem with yo-yo dieting is that weight isn't the only aspect of your health that is being affected! This type of dieting increases your blood pressure, enlarges your heart, damages your kidneys, increases your abdominal fat deposits **and** promotes ENORMOUS weight gain

METABOLIC SET POINT

Your Metabolic Set Point is when your body is used to being a certain weight. When your body is at this point, it doesn't want to change or stray very far from it.

This is an example of what's called your Metabolic Set Point:

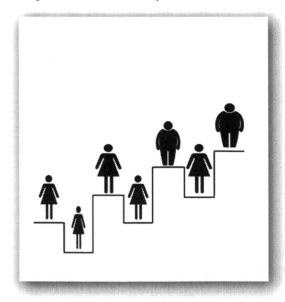

Here is the story of Jane.

Jane is 20 years old, weighs 135lbs and looks great! She saw this super-model on TV that weighs 105lbs so she thought that she needed to lose weight until she looked like that model. So she went on her first fad diet. She ate fake foods, MRPs, had tons of nutrient deficiencies and was missing pleasure from food. But she made it to 100lbs. The next thing you know, she was STARVING. Her hunger hormones were through the roof. She lost a bunch of muscle and she said, "Forget this, I can't do this anymore. I'm starving!" Provided with no education, she started to eat like she used to again. She quickly went back to her start weight and actually gained even MORE weight. Now she's 180lbs. At this point, she can't stand the way she looks and tells herself, "What was I thinking? I looked great at 135lbs, and now I'm 180lbs! I'll just go on another diet." She watched a show that told her to take a pill, not eat breakfast or lunch, and fell into another fad diet. She was able to get back down to her original weight of 135lbs, but she wasn't able to sustain it. Her hunger hormones went through the roof again and she lost muscle mass. This led her to go up and up and up. The next thing you know, her Metabolic Set Point is over 200lbs! This is all because of fad diet after fad diet that "remodeled" her Metabolic Set Point higher each time.

*Remember, muscle is the #1 driver of your metabolism – each time you go on these fad diets you lose lean muscle, essentially remodeling your Metabolic Set Point.

These fad diets really just end up leaving you with:

- More fat
- Less muscle
- No education

BREAKING THE CYCLE

So when you are looking at food, you should ask yourself:

- How was the food grown?
- How was the food processed?
- How old is the food?
- Does it have the "sum of the whole food?"

Remember that **quality** is #1 when you are looking at food! You should be concentrating mainly on your plant-based nutrition. Vegetables are going to be the biggest focus for your program. I can say it a thousand times: it's not a sprint - it's a marathon. When you get to the end, you are finally going to see lifetime results!

*The Rant: With so many fad diets all around us, it's difficult not to fall victim to them when receiving short-term results – keep in mind that taking it slow and steady will lead to permanent results.

Lifestyle Scale	DESCRIPTION
Serving Size 1 Person Makes 1 Lifetime Result	**Difficulty** – Making **better** choices is the hardest part of eating out.
Grade Per Person	
Grade	
Grade*	
Difficulty 3	**Time to Implement** – You make **better** choices one day at a time.
Time to Implement 1 Day	**Importance** – Making better choices at a **restaurant** will help in all **aspects** of health.
Importance 5	
*Amount is based off of the average person. Your personal results may be higher or lower depending on your specific needs.	

25

Dining out

Okay, so when you think about eating healthy and staying fit, you might think that you're going to have to give up all the pleasures in your life and lock yourself in your house with a stalk of celery and some apples. It's totally not true. You can still enjoy the pleasures in life like going out to eat, but you have to be ready to make SMARTER decisions. Living a healthy lifestyle can provide you with some of the best tasting foods out there!

WE ALL HAVE OBLIGATIONS

While the ideal is to avoid restaurants at all costs, that's not a reality. Whether it's a business luncheon, birthday party or a Friday date night, we all have obligations in life that we have to attend to, and most of these will eventually involve going out to eat. The good part is that restaurants are finally starting to "get it" and put nutritious and body-friendly foods on their menus. Still, not every restaurant creates well-balanced meals on their menus, so you'll need to watch out for certain "trigger words" so that you can make better decisions about the food you order.

FOODS ARE DECEIVING

You might think that salad, chicken or soup would be okay, but restaurants have found a way to make even these options some of the worst choices on their menus by doctoring them up with hidden sugars, trans fats, industrial seed oils, unhealthy cooking tactics and more. Restaurants are notorious for adding ingredients to foods that make them more delicious, though not necessarily more nutritious.

WATCH OUT FOR HIDDEN SUGAR

How can you hide sugars from the consumers? Aside from being found in main dishes and desserts (obviously), most dressings are filled with sugar and unhealthy fat to make them taste better as well. These sugars are also found in your ketchup, barbecue sauce, spaghetti sauce, cranberry sauce, breaded dishes and hamburgers!

Did I just say hamburgers? Yes, that wasn't a typo. Restaurants use sugar to reduce meat shrinkage, giving you a larger looking portion when the dish hits the table.

STEER CLEAR FROM INDUSTRIAL SEED OILS

Industrial seed oils cause havoc in your body just the same as sugar does by increasing inflammation. Remembering which oils are healthy or healthier can be confusing. Only SOME oils are good for the body, like **coconut oil**, **cold-pressed extra-virgin olive oil**, **flaxseed oil** and the healthy **omega-3 oils** found in fish like wild-caught salmon. Most restaurants, on the other hand, use cheaper oils like safflower, sunflower, corn, cottonseed, sesame, peanut and soybean oil. All of these oils are found in your chips, crackers, dressings and restaurant foods.

TRANS FAT WARNING

Trans fats are the unhealthy and far less expensive alternative to olive oil. Many restaurants use cheaper fat like Crisco lard to cook their food, which puts hydrogenated fats in your fried appetizers, French fries, cookies, cakes and more.

BAD TRIGGER WORDS

Some "Bad Trigger Words" on menus that you should avoid include anything that's:

- Battered
- Buttery
- Creamy
- Cheesy
- Thick
- Smothered
- Glazed

Additionally, avoid heavy creams, special sauces and gravies, which are all loaded with fat. You'll be making **a better, healthier choice** by asking your server to remove these from your order.

SUBSTITUTE THE BAD STARCHES

If you're somewhat physically active, you might wonder about pasta. I can tell you that most sauces are loaded with unhealthy fats, and most pasta is highly processed, losing its valuable nutritional properties! You should avoid any breads, breaded items, mashed potatoes, pasta and loaded rice that accompany most meals because your body easily stores these refined carbohydrates as fat. Remember that **sweet potatoes and red potatoes are a great substitute for any white potato option**. However, stay away from mashed potatoes, because they have hidden fats and are higher in sugar. Additionally, when you mash a potato, you start the digestive process, and the hotter the mashed potatoes are, the faster they digest. When you digest food too quickly, your blood sugar spikes, which causes a downward stream of negative hormonal effects.

TAKE THE BREAD AWAY, PLEASE!

One part of going out to eat that people struggle with is sitting at your table looking at that warm bread basket that is calling out, "Come on, throw some butter on me and eat me before I get cold." If that bread basket is tempting you too much, don't be afraid to ask your server to remove it from the table right when you sit down. Furthermore, don't add any butter to your meals as this only adds unhealthy fats and unwanted calories to your food.

EVADE THE APPETIZERS

Most people start off their meal with an appetizer, but you should actually skip appetizers altogether, even if they have something seemingly healthy in them like artichokes. I say this because they're usually filled with unhealthy trans fats and are one of the more deceiving types of foods that you see at restaurants.

How deceiving you ask? Let's take those artichokes I mentioned for example. An artichoke heart salad from a restaurant can be just about 155 calories without a major amount of dressing. Not bad. Now compare that to artichoke dip from your favorite chain restaurant, which contains 1,510 calories, 99 grams of fat and 125 grams of carbohydrates. That's enough fat for almost two days!

BE MINDFUL AT BUFFETS

Buffets are often one of the worst options for eating out, but they're big at family parties, weddings and other events, and therefore unavoidable. First off, you need to resist the temptation to overeat in order to get the best bang for your buck. The fact of the matter is that the extra calories are going to force you to work harder to reach your health and fat-loss goals. Of course, there **are** some healthy – or at least **healthier** – options!

Hit the salad bar FIRST, but look out for low-fat or fat-free dressings since they have hidden sugar, bad fats and even processed GMO soy, which are all linked to a bunch of diseases[1].

MAKE THE BETTER CHOICE

Choose as many veggies as you can and complement them with a **small amount** of lean protein such as chicken, turkey, beans or a **small amount** of nuts. However, don't eat the skin of chicken, turkey or duck because it's **filled with fat**. Additionally, steer clear from any carb-filled meal such as pasta or rice that could be mixed in with your meats. Stay away from soups that are cream- or sherry-based, and don't have anything that contains pasta, white potatoes or white rice. Instead, look for soups that have beans, low sodium broth, lean meats, brown rice and, of course, veggies! Dessert is a very tricky part of eating out. If you must have a dessert, get fresh fruit. Or, better yet, make your own dessert at home, which is not only cheaper, but you can replace unhealthy added sugars and fats with healthier stevia or coconut oil, and it will still taste good!

DON'T FORGET TO DRINK WATER

Numerous studies have shown that drinking 1-2 glasses of water prior to eating your meal can curb your appetite so that you consume fewer calories because water gives your body a sense of fullness[2]. I always recommend drinking 16 oz. (two glasses) of water prior to going out to eat because it normally takes about a half-hour to flush out your hunger hormones, so you won't feel like you're starving by the time you have your meal!

Calories don't come just from the foods that you eat, but from the liquids that you drink as well! Water contains zero calories, so you have nothing to worry about there. However, sweetened teas, sodas, beers, wines and hard liquors all contain liquid calories. If you don't enjoy the taste of water, or you're just in the mood for something a little more flavorful, consider enjoying sparkling water with a lemon – it'll save you a lot of calories.

GOOD TRIGGER WORDS

Now that we've established all the bad things to keep an eye out for, let's take a look at some "Good Trigger Words" to look for, including:

- Broiled
- Steamed
- Baked
- Roasted
- Light
- Fresh
- Grilled
- Sautéed in olive oil

PLAN AHEAD

You can search most restaurants' menus online before going out so that you'll know ahead of time what's healthy to eat even before you get there. Not only will you avoid making a poor decision by feeling rushed, but it will also cut down on the amount of time it takes to get your food. Who doesn't love that idea?

If you know ahead of time, plan your day around your going out meal. Have a light lunch if you're going to eat out at dinnertime, but don't skip meals. If it's more of a last minute decision, eat a light snack like some veggies or a handful of nuts to help satisfy your hunger before you even leave your house. Going out to eat hungry is only tempting yourself to order unhealthy or less healthy meals. After putting in so much hard work throughout the week you don't want to face a major setback because of just one meal.

TAKE CONTROL

Furthermore, request your dressing on the side so that YOU can control how much is added to your food. Try dunking your fork in the dressing to coat it with sauce **before** picking up any veggies in your salad. You can also skip the dressing entirely and just squeeze a lemon over your food to reduce your fat calories. No more soggy veggies!

Eliminate croutons, cheese, bacon bits and fried onions from your salads since these can add a lot of needless calories. Look for salads with beans, fruits, tomatoes, sliced carrots, cucumbers, snap peas and other fresh veggies. Avoid iceberg lettuce, which is low in nutrients, and look for spinach, romaine or any other mixed green to act as the base of your salad.

Substitute a side of fries or battered onion rings for a house salad or mixed vegetables.

PRACTICE YOUR PORTION CONTROL

Most restaurants' portions are enough for two, so remember to pay attention to your portion control! You can save on calories and money when you split your plate of food with someone you're dining with or just as good, take half of it home in a doggie bag. Make it a point to pause when you're halfway through your meal to sit back and ask yourself if you're still hungry. You might be amazed that most of the time the answer is "no." If you're not feeling confident that you'll be able to stop yourself halfway through your meal, don't worry – ask your server to have half your food wrapped up "to go" when you put your order in.

ENJOY YOUR FOOD!

As always, eating slowly is crucial. Not only will you enjoy the food thoroughly and be more likely to chew properly, but you'll also feel fuller after eating less because it takes your brain about 20 minutes to notice that you're full[3]. Concentrating on conversation with whoever you're eating with and putting your fork down between bites to sip on water are good ways to pace yourself.

GOING OUT LATE?

If you're going out later at night, avoid carbs and alcohol as both can block your body from burning fat. Try not to eat within the three hours leading up to your bedtime, but if you do need to eat something, then choose green veggies or mainly green veggies with a small portion of a lean protein!

*The Rant: Making smarter decisions when dining out will help you attain your fitness goals – all while feeling satisfied by still being able to take part in the activity of dining out.

Appendix A

Alkalinity

You may have heard of alkalinity before, but what does it have to do with nutrition, and especially fat loss? Everything alive wants to remain in homeostasis, which is where your body is at its most properly functioning state. For human beings, our point of homeostasis is anywhere between 7.35 and 7.45 on the pH scale, leaving us slightly more alkaline (basic).

WHAT DOES IT DO?

When we keep our body in an alkaline state, our red blood cells get supercharged with a negative charge, which keeps them from sticking together and allows them to transport oxygen more efficiently. In an acidic state, our blood's negative charge wears away to leave the positive core exposed, leading to red blood cells sticking to each other, thus slowing the process.

Unfortunately, the average adult ingests around 80 percent acidic foods and 20 percent alkaline. Believe it or not, you should be the exact opposite of this: 80 percent alkaline and 20 percent acidic. You can achieve this balance through plant-based nutrition, meaning vegetables and fruits. Notice that I listed vegetables first. It's because vegetables are going to provide you with the most fiber and nutrients while still remaining low in sugar.

LOOK FOR THESE

Some vegetables that you should be looking to ingest include:

- Peas
- Lima beans
- Artichokes
- Cabbage
- Carrots
- Radishes
- Watercress
- Spinach
- Turnips
- Brussels sprouts
- Cucumbers

When thinking fruit, look to ingest:

- Lemon (acidic, but after ingested it becomes alkaline in your bloodstream)
- Watermelon
- Avocados
- Grapefruit
- Pears
- Apples
- Bananas
- Cantaloupe
- Grapes

To a lesser degree other alkaline foods include:

- Almonds
- Pine nuts
- Cashews

- Walnuts
- Flaxseed
- Sesame seed
- Brown rice
- Quinoa

STAY AWAY FROM THESE

Acidic foods you should avoid include:

- Hamburgers
- Hot dogs
- Lunch meat
- Cookies
- Alcohol
- Soda
- White bread, or any bread for that matter
- Cheese and other dairy products
- Noodles
- Coffee
- Processed food

Appendix B

How do sweeteners rank?

Although all sweeteners taste sweet, different sweeteners have different effects on your body. There are definitely some sweeteners that rank on the low end of the spectrum compared to others.

The worst sweeteners:

- Sucralose (AKA Splenda)
- Aspartame (AKA NutraSweet)

A close second to the worst:

- High fructose corn syrup
- Fruit juice concentrate
- Agave nectar

Third worst:

- White sugar
- Brown sugar
- Molasses

Better:

- Coconut sugar
- Raw honey

The best:

- Xylitol
- Stevia

Even though **xylitol** and **stevia** are the best, you should still only use them sparingly. No matter how you put it, a high amount of any kind of sugar can still lead to problems down the road.

Sucralose, better known as **Splenda**, is created from chlorinating sugar. This chlorine consumption can affect your immune system and lead to a damaged thyroid.

Aspartame, better known as **NutraSweet**, is another non-natural sweetener. It has been linked with epilepsy, brain tumors and Parkinson's disease. It has also been shown to damage your digestive system.

High fructose corn syrup is processed from genetically modified corn starch. This type of sugar is extremely high on the glycemic index.

Fruit juice concentrate is a processed juice from fruits such as white grapes and oranges. Fruit juice concentrate has been processed so much that it provides your body with few nutrients, but leaves you with all the sugar to rush into your liver.

Agave nectar is a food that has been marketed as "healthy" from big companies. Even though this is a natural sweetener, it can contain up to

90% fructose, which has to be broken down by your liver and usually leads to fat storage in the long-run.

*High fructose corn syrup, fruit juice concentrate and agave nectar must be processed in your liver. They bypass the brain's satiety switch causing your body to overeat.

White sugar is typically made from sugarcane, beets or corn. In more recent years, it is processed usually from genetically modified crops, which provide your body with no nutrients or minerals.

Even though many people claim that **brown sugar** is much better than white, it is really just white sugar mixed with molasses to give it that brown look and sticky consistency.

Molasses is a byproduct of the pressing of sugarcane.

Coconut sugar is made from the juices of coconut palm blossoms. The plant's nectar is heated until it caramelizes, then is ground into a powder.

Raw honey is made from bees that have retrieved nectar from plants. The combination of their enzymes in their stomachs transforms the nectar into what we know as honey, which they spread around their hives to dry out.

Xylitol is a sugar alcohol, which means that it is very low on the glycemic index. Even though it is found in nature, it can still negatively affect your bowels if ingested in high quantities.

Stevia is a naturally-occurring sweetener taken from the Stevia rebaudiana plant, which is found mostly in South America. It is shown that Stevia is up to 300 times sweeter than normal sugar **and** has zero calories!

Because of this combination, I recommend substituting Stevia for any type of sugar currently in your diet.

*For additional information and references visit www.sweettoothtruth.com

Appendix C

Glycemic index

WARNING: The Glycemic Index is not a health scale. Therefore, I do not recommend following it. However, since many people use it in the health industry, it is still important for you to understand it.

Each food has been ranked on the glycemic index, which shows how fast or slow food is digested and turned into usable energy.

The **lower** the glycemic index, the slower the food will be digested, which means it's less likely to be stored as fat because your metabolism will be elevated throughout the day. Foods low on the glycemic index include complex carbohydrates (sweet potatoes, rice bread, quinoa, etc.) healthy fats (avocados, mixed nuts, olive oil, etc.), and quality proteins (grass-fed meats, organic eggs, wild-caught fish, etc.).

The **higher** the glycemic index, on the other hand, the faster that food can be digested, causing an immediate spike of blood sugar, which leads to excess energy in the bloodstream as well as an increase in fat storage. Foods high on the glycemic index include simple carbs (refined sugar, white bread, candy, etc.) and processed food-like products (chips, convenience bars, etc.), all of which slow your metabolism down.

References

Chapter 1

1. Orden C.L Etal. Prevalence of childhood and adult obesity in the United States. 2014 Journal of the America Medical Association, 311(8), 806-814

2. Pratley, R., Nicklas, B., Rubin, M., Miller, J., Smith, A., Smith, M., Hurley, B., & Goldberg, A. (1994). Strength training increases resting metabolic rate and norepinephrine levels in healthy 50- to 65-yr-old men. Journal of Applied Physiology, 76, 133-137

Chapter 2

1. American Academy of Environmental Medicine. Genetically Modified Foods. Availably at: http://www.aaemonline.org/gmopost.html

2. The Nation. Twenty-Six Countries Ban GMO- Why Won't the US? Availably at: http://www.thenation.com/blog/176863/twenty-six-countries-ban-gmos-why-wont-us

Chapter 3

1. Zimmermann M. Burgerstein's Handbook of Nutrition: Micronutrients in the Prevention and Therapy of Disease. New York: Thieme; 2001.

2. Ludwig DS. Examining the Health Effects of Fructose. JAMA. 2013;310(1):33-34

3. Berg JM etal. Biochemistry. 5th edition. New York ; W H Freeman; 2002. Available at: http://www.ncbi.nlm.nih.gov/books/NBK22545/

4. National Foundation for Celiac Awareness. What is Celiac Disease? Available at: http://www.celiaccentral.org/newlydiagnosed/What-is-Celiac-Disease/1103/

5. Phytic Acid.Org. Phytic acid, Tips For Consumers From Food Science. Available at: http://www.phyticacid.org/

6. Hyman M. The Blood Sugar Solution. New York: Hachette Book Group; 2012

7. John and Ocean Robbins. Living The Food Revolution. Available at: http://foodrevolution.org/

8. Sizer FS, Whitney E. Nutrition: Concepts & Controversies. Belmont, CA: Wadsworth; 2011.

9. Flegal KM. Epidemiologic aspects of overweight and obesity in the United States. Physiology & Behavior. Volume 86, issue 5, 15 December 2005, pages 599-602

10. Siri-Tarino PW etal. Meta-analysis of prospective cohort studies evaluating the association of saturated fat with cardiovascular disease. Am J Clin Nutr. 2010 Mar; 91 (3): 535-546.

11. GB HealthWatch. Omega-3 : Omega-6 balance. Available: http://www.gbhealthwatch.com/Science-Omega3-Omega6.php

12. Kresser C. 9 Steps to perfect health. PDF available at http://chriskresser.com/

Chapter 4

1. Connecticut College News. Student-faculty research suggests Oreos can be compared to drugs of abuse in lab rats. 10/15/13 available at: http://www.conncoll.edu/news/news-archive/2013/student-faculty-research-suggests-oreos-can-be-compared-to-drugs-of-abuse-in-lab-rats.htm#.VM7FQmTF90I

2. Hyman M. The Blood Sugar Solution. New York: Hachette Book Group; 2012

3. Medical daily. Opinion: nutrition facts labels may soon include added sugar info; food companies protest despite risk of obese, disease America.

Available at: http://www.medicaldaily.com/opinion-nutrition-facts-labels-may-soon-include-added-sugar-info-food-companies-308834

Chapter 5
1. Organic Consumers Association. All About Organics. Available at: https://www.organicconsumers.org/organlink
2. Environmental Working Group. Dirty Dozen and the Clean fifteen. Available at: http://www.ewg.org/

Chapter 7
1.Dr. T Colin Campbell and Thomas M. Campbell II. The China Study: The Most Comprehensive Study of Nutrition Ever Conducted and the Startling Implications for Diet, Weight Loss and Long Term Health. BenZBella Books, 6440 N. Central Expressway, Dallas, TX 75206
2.Chan JM, Etal. Dairy Products, Calcium, and Vitamin D and Risk of Prostate Cancer. Epidemiological Review 23 (2001), 87-92.
3. Davis W. Wheat Belly Total Health: The Ultimate Grain-Free Health and Weight-Loss Life Plan. Special Market Department, Rodale Inc. 733 Third Avenue, New York, NY 10017
4. University of Wisconsin. Teaching Modules & Patient Handouts. Available at: https://www.fammed.wisc.edu/integrative/modules

Chapter 8
1. Backhed F, Ding H, Wang T, Hooper LV, Koh GY, Nagy A, Semenkovich CF, Gordon JI. The gut microbiota as an environmental factor that regulates fat storage. Proc Natl Acad Sci U S A.2004 Nov 2:101(44):15718-23. http://www.ncbi.nlm.nih.gov/pmc/articles/PMC524219/
2.Vijay_KumarM et al. Metabolic syndrome and altered gut microbiota in mice lacking Toll-like receptor 5. Science. 2010 April 9;328(5975):228-31. doi: http://www.ncbi.nlm.nih.gov/pubmed/20203013
3. David, Marc. The Slow Down Diet: Eating for Pleasure, Energy, and Weight Loss. 2005

Chapter 12
1. Olshansky Sj. A potential decline in life expectancy in the United States in the 21st century. N Engl J Med.2005 Mar 17;352(11): 1138-45. http://www.ncbi.nlm.nih.gov/pubmed/10891514
2. Wolever T etal. Second_meal effects:low-gycemic-index foods eaten at dinner improve subsequent breakfast glycemic response. Am J Clin Nutr 1988;48:1041-7
3. Katch F, Katch V, McArdle WD. Exercise Physiology: Nutrition, Energy, and Human Performance. Baltimore, MD: Lippincott Williams & Wilkins, a Wolters Kluwer business; 2010.

Chapter 13
1. Sizer FS, Whitney E. Nutrition: Concepts & Controversies. Belmont, CA: Wadsworth; 2011.
2. Natural Resources Defense Council. Bottle Water, Pure Drink or Pure Hype? Available at: http://www.nrdc.org/water/drinking/bw/bwinx.asp
3. Natural Resources Defense Council. Phthalates. Available at: http://www.nrdc.org/living/chemicalindex/phthalates.asp?gclid=CKTF4vLN6cICFY_m7Aod9xsA1g
4. Burke L, Deakin V. Clinical Sports Nutrition. Australia: McGraw-Hill Australia Pty Ltd; 2010.
5. Katch F, Katch V, McArdle WD. Exercise Physiology: Nutrition, Energy, and Human Performance. Baltimore, MD: Lippincott Williams & Wilkins, a Wolters Kluwer business; 2010.
6. Hyman M. The Blood Sugar Solution. New York: Hachette Book Group; 2012.
7. Simon BR etal. Artificial sweeteners stimulate adipogenesis and suppress lipolysis independently of sweet taste receptors. J Biol Chem Nov 8;288(45):32475-89
8. Swithers SE, Davidson TL. A role for sweet taste: calorie predictive relations in energy regulation by rats. Behav Neurosci 2008 Feb; 122(1):161-73

9. Langton N. How much red wine do you need to get enough resveratrol? Updated article August 16, 2013 available at: http://www.livestrong.com/article/411745-how-much-red-wine-do-you-need-to-get-enough-resveratrol/

Chapter 14
1. Burke L, Deakin V. Clinical Sports Nutrition. Australia: McGraw-Hill Australia Pty Ltd; 2010.
2. McArdle WD, Katch FI, Katch VL. Exercise Physiology Nutritional. Energy, and Human Performance seventh, edition. 2010

Chapter 15
1. Lee, I. Physical Activity. The Lancet Published:july 18, 2012 available at: http://www.thelancet.com/series/physical-activity
2. Praag HV. Neurogenesis and Exercise: Past and Future Directions. June 2008, Volume 10, Issue 2, pp 128-140
3.Menshikova EV etal. Effects of Exercise on Mitochondrial Content and Function in Aging Human Skeletal Muscle. J Gerontol A Biol Sci Med Sci. 2006 Jun; 61(6); 534-540.
4. Holloszy JO. Regulation by exercise of skeletal muscle content of mitochondria and GLUT4. J Physiol Pharmacol 2008 Dec;59 Suppl 7:5-18.
5. ACE Personal Training Manual. San Diego, CA: American Council on Exercise; 2010.
6. McArdle WD, Katch FI, Katch VL. Exercise Physiology Nutritional. Energy, and Human Performance seventh, edition. 2010
7. Wolfe RR. Metabolic interactions between glucose and fatty acids in human. Am J Clin Nutr
8. Katch F, Katch V, McArdle WD. Exercise Physiology: Nutrition, Energy, and Human Performance. Baltimore, MD: Lippincott Williams & Wilkins, a Wolters Kluwer business; 2010.
9. Burke L, Deakin V. Clinical Sports Nutrition. Australia: McGraw-Hill Australia Pty Ltd; 2010.

Chapter 16
1. Rogers, S A - Using organic acids to diagnose and manage recalcitrant patients. Alternative therapy, Jul/Aug 2006, Vol. 12 No4.
2. Perera, F P - molecular epidemiology: insight into cancer susceptibility, risk assessment and prevention. J Natl Cancer Inst. 1996;88(8):496-509, April 17, 1996
3. Samman S etal. Fatty acid composition of certified organic, conventional and omega 3 eggs

Chapter 18
1. Haidt J. The Happiness Hypothesis Finding Modern Truth in Ancient Wisdom. Available at: http://www.happinesshypothesis.com/buy.html
2. Moore K. ZEN 12 user guide. Program available at http://www.zen12.com/
3. Harris B. Thresholds of the Mind, Your Personal Roadmap to Success, Happiness and Contentment. Program available at: https://www.center-pointe.com/v2/
4. McGonigal K. The Willpower Instinct: How Self-Control Works, Why If Matters, and What You Can Do to Get More of It. Available at: http://kellymcgonigal.com/willpowerinstinct/
5. Holzel, B K etal. Mindfulness practice leads to increases in regional brain gray matter density. Psychiatry Res. Jan 30, 2011
6. Bhasin MK etal. Relaxation Response Induces Temporal Transcriptome Changes in Energy Metabolism, Insulin Secretion and Inflammatory Pathways. PLOS one May 01, 2013

Chapter 19
1. CDC Website. Insufficient Sleep Is a Public Health Epidemic. Available at: http://www.cdc.gov/features/dssleep/
2.World Health Organization website. The breast cancer conundrum. Available at: http://www.who.int/bulletin/volumes/91/9/13-020913/en/

3. Institute of Medicine website. Sleep Disorders and Sleep Deprivation:An Unmet Public Health Problem. Available at: http://www.iom.edu/Reports/2006/Sleep-Disorders-and-Sleep-Deprivation-An-Unmet-Public-Health-Problem.aspx

4. National Sleep Foundation. Website: http://sleepfoundation.org/

5. CNN Interactive. Lack of sleep American's top health problem, doctors say. Available at: http://www.cnn.com/HEALTH/9703/17/nfm/sleep.deprivation/

6. The Western Diet and Lifestyle and Diseases of Civilization. Available at: http://www.dovepress.com/the-western-diet-and-lifestyle-and-diseases-of-civilization-peer-reviewed-article-RRCC.

7. Coping with excessive sleepiness. 10 Things to Hate About Sleep Loss. Available at: http://www.webmd.com/sleep-disorders/excessive-sleepiness-10/10-results-sleep-loss?page=2

8. Broussard JL etal. Impaired Insulin Signaling in Human Adipocytes After Experimental Sleep Restriction: A Randomized, Crossover Sudy. American College of Physicians 16 October 2012, Vol 157.

9. McCusker RR etal. Caffeine Content of Decaffeinated Coffee. Journal of Analytical Toxicology, Vol 30, October 2006.

Chapter 20

1. WebMD. The effects of Stress on Your Body. Available at: http://www.webmd.com/balance/stress-management/effects-of-stress-on-your-body

2. Hanson R. Hardwiring Happiness The New Brian Science of Contentment, Clam, and Confidence. Book available at: http://www.rickhanson.net/books/hardwiring-happiness/

3. Aschbacher K etal. Good stress, bad stress and oxidative stress: insight from anticipatory cortisol reactivity. Pychoneuroendocrinology . 2013 Sep;38(9):1698-708

4. Freedman DS, Dietz WH, Srinivas SR, Berenson GS. The relation of overweight to cardiovascular risk factors among children and adolescents:

the Bogalusa Heart Study. *Pediatrics* 1999 Jun; 103(6 Pt1): 1175-82. Available at: http://www.ncbi.nlm.nih.gov/pubmed/10353925 6/3/2013
5. Zimmermann M. *Burgerstein's Handbook of Nutrition: Micronutrients in the Prevention and Therapy of Disease*. New York: Thieme; 2001

Chapter 21
1. Shimoff M. Happy for No Reason seven steps to being Happy from the Inside Out. Book available at: http://www.happyfornoreason.com/bookbonuses

Chapter 22
1. Bralley JA, Lord RS. *Laboratory Evaluations For Integrative and Functional Medicine*. Duluth, GA: Metametrix Institute; 2012.
2. Baker, Sidney MD. Website available at: http://www.healthgrades.com/physician/dr-sidney-baker-xmrnh Quote from notes "Therapeutic Nutrition Review: GI, Detox, Inflammation" Sylvia H Regalla MD, MSACN
3. Liska D PH.D. The Role of Detoxification in the Prevention of Chronic Degenerative Disease. ANSR-Applied Nutritional Science Reports Rev. 8/05
4. Jones etal. Environmental pollution and diabetes: a neglected association. Lancet Jan 26;371.

Chapter 23
1. The Healing Effect Movie. Available at: http://thehealingeffect.com
2. Calton, J. Could Micronutrient Deficiency be a missing link in the fight against overweight/obesity. JAAIM fall 2010 PDF available at: http://www.aaimedicine.com/pdf/jaaim/news-letters/JM10-3fall.pdf
3. Simopoulus AP. The importance of the ratio of omega-6/omega-3 fatty acids. Biomed Pharmacother. 2002 Oct; 56(8): 365-79. availible at: http://www.ncbi.nlm.nih.gov/pubmed/12442909
4. Aggarwal BB, Krishnan S, Guha S. *Inflammation, Lifestyle, and Chronic Disease: The Silent Link*. Boca Raton, FL: Taylor & Francis Group; 2012.

5. Groff JL, Gropper SS, Smith JL. *Advanced Nutrition and Human Metabolism.* Belmont, CA: Wadsworth; 2009.

Chapter 24
1. Wing RR and Hill JO. Successful Weight Loss Maintenance. Annual Review of Nutrition Vol. 21 323-342
2. American Cancer Society. Lycopene. Article available at: http://www.cancer.org/treatment/treatmentsandsideeffects/ complementaryandalternativemedicine/dietandnutrition/lycopene
3. Brownell KD Etal. The effects of repeated cycles of weight loss and regain in rats. Physiol Behav. 1986 Oct;38(4):459-64.

Chapter 25
1. Mercola.com. 19 Studies Link GMO Foods to Organ Disruption. Article available at: http://articles.mercola.com/sites/articles/archive/2011/04/27/19 -studies-link-gmo-foods-to-organ-disruption.aspx April 27, 2011
2. American Chemical Society. Drink water to curb weight gain? Clinical trial confirms effectiveness of simple appetite control method. Article available at: http://www.sciencedaily.com/releases/2010/08/100823142929. htm August 23, 2010
3. MacDonald A from Harvard Health. Why eating slowly may help you feel full faster. Article available at: http://www.health.harvard.edu/blog/ why-eating-slowly-may-help-you-feel-full-faster-20101019605 October 19, 2010

FRANKFORT FREE LIBRARY
123 Frankfort St.
Frankfort, NY 13340
(315) 894-9611

5/2/15

15 —

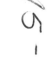

Made in the USA
Middletown, DE
10 June 2015